Praise for *Addiction &*

"Barb Rogers knew grief, inside and out. How lucky for all the readers of her many books that she left us with this last one. Grieving is a natural state of life, and Rogers shares with clarity what it looks like and how to grow beyond it. She knew the path well. Now it's our turn to grieve her loss."
—Karen Casey, author of *Change Your Mind and Your Life will Follow*

"Barb Rogers left us a wonder-filled testament on how healing and transforming emotions allows us to celebrate the fullness of life."
—Mary Cook, MA, RAS, author of *Grace Lost and Found: From Addictions and Compulsions to Satisfaction and Serenity*

"Barb Rogers has left us many wonderful gifts, and this book is clearly one of the most valuable. Those of us suffering from addiction never learned how to cope with feelings, especially feelings of loss, disappointment, and grief. Our solution was to avoid our pain by numbing our feelings. This was self-destructive. In *Addiction and Grief,* Barb guides us on a journey of self-discovery that teaches us healthier ways of coping with these painful feelings. Please read this book; it will help you find emotional sobriety and strengthen your recovery program. Barb, you will be missed but will live on in our hearts in your wonderful writings."

—Allen Berger, PhD, psychologist and author of *12 Stupid Things That Mess Up Recovery* and *12 Smart Things to Do When the Booze and Drugs are Gone*

"Much of recovery is about dealing with loss. Addicts drink, gamble, and drug away the most precious things life has to offer while in their disease and then need to come to terms with all the destruction they've caused in sobriety. In this marvelous book, Barb Rogers offers gentle insight into the roots of this grief and provides clear tools for airing out the past misdeeds and going forward into the sunshine. A must read for anyone interested in quality recovery."

—Elizabeth Engstrom, author of *York's Moon*

"This book is a practical touchstone in the often shadowy world of ancient fears that silently haunt the recovered life. Hold it closely."

—William Alexander, author of *Ordinary Recovery: Mindfulness, Addiction, and the Path of Lifelong Sobriety*

"Barb Rogers says, 'Grief is the last stronghold of addicts.' She encourages the reader to face their fear, deal with the anger, and heal the grief. Rogers passionately shares her personal journey through her own lifetime of losses and grief which eventually led her to true inner peace. Thank you, Barb Rogers, for leaving our planet with such a wise and empowering book!"

—Barbara Joy, author of *Easy Does It, Mom* and *Moms to Moms: Parenting Wisdom from Moms in Recovery*

Addiction
& Grief

Also by Barb Rogers

If I Die Before I Wake: A Memoir of Drinking and Recovery

Clutter No More: 12 Steps to Freeing Your Life from Your Stuff

12 Steps That Can Save Your Life: Real-Life Stories from People Who Are Walking the Walk

Keep It Simple and Sane: Freeing Yourself from Addictive Thinking

Clutter Junkie No More: Stepping Up to Recovery

Costumes, Accessories, Props, and Stage Illusions Made Easy

Twenty-Five Words: How the Serenity Prayer Can Save Your Life

Pray for Today (Just Try This)

Simply Happy Every Day (Just Try This)

Feng Shui in a Day (Just Try This)

Mystic Glyphs: An Oracle Based on Native American Symbols

Instant Period Costumes: How to Make Classic Costumes from Cast-Off Clothing

Costuming Made Easy: How to Make Theatrical Costumes from Cast-Off Clothing

Addiction
& Grief

Letting Go of Fear,
Anger, and Addiction

Barb Rogers

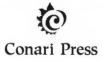

Conari Press

First published in 2011 by
Conari Press, an imprint of
Red Wheel/Weiser, LLC
665 Third Street, Suite 400
San Francisco, CA 94107
www.redwheelweiser.com

ISBN: 978-1-57324-516-6

Library of Congress Cataloging-in-Publication Data

is available upon request.

Cover design by Jim Warner

Cover photograph: Fog over a lake at sunrise, Scott Lake,
Willamette National Forest, Oregon, USA. Copyright © Don
Paulson Photography/Purestock/SuperStock

Typeset by Stan Info

Printed in the United States of America
MAL
10 9 8 7 6 5 4 3 2 1
The paper used in this publication meets the
minimum requirements of the American National Standard
for Information Sciences—Permanence of Paper for
Printed Library Materials Z39.48-1992 (R1997).

Publisher's Note

Barb Rogers, with whom we published several books, died suddenly in early 2011 as this book was being edited. Over the years, Barb became a friend as well as a colleague. Her ready humor and big heart were evident in her interactions with all of us.

In this book, Barb wrote, "You never know how much time you have on this earth, so don't let the moments slip by as you agonize over past experiences or fantasize about tomorrow. This moment and this day are yours, and what you do with them is your choice."

Barb, may this gift you've left behind move people to make the choices to leave grief, fear, and anger in the past and live fully in the present, one day at a time. We are grateful and proud to be publishing this book.

—Jan Johnson, Publisher, Conari Press

In memory of my brother-in-law,
Don Rogers of Wrights Corner, Illinois,
who will be remembered for his big heart,
gentle nature, and absolutely wicked sense of
humor. He will be missed by all who loved him.
And to Calvin Gordon, the miracle dog we
nearly lost this year, and his lovely
companion, the lovely Nikki.

Contents

Acknowledgments 13

Introduction 15

Grieve It Forward 21

Living Proof 29

The Storm Within 35

The "G" List 41

Whispers and Screams 51

Excuse Me? I'm Addicted 61

Strange Packages 67

Frenemies 73

Recycle 79

Balance Sheet 85

Who Loves Ya, Baby? 91

Good Grief 101

All or Nothing 109

Letting Go 115

Fear, Anger, Grief, Addiction 117

Celebrate 133

Dance on Life 139

Acknowledgments

My gratitude to Jan Johnson, Michael Kerber, and the entire staff of Red Wheel/Weiser Books and Conari Press for giving me the opportunity to do what I love. For every person whose life is touched by one of my books, it is your hands that make it possible.

To all the friends of Bill W. who are too many to name that have crossed through my life, leaving their bits of wisdom that I might have the life I have today, I thank you.

A special thank you to Armondo Casas of Congress, Arizona, who, through my challenge with physical problems over the past few years, has been my inspiration. I have watched in awe as you handled your own problems with grace and dignity, and it gave me hope. And, to Dr. William Firth, my absolutely favorite doctor and my friend.

I could not have gotten through this last year without the help of Susie Tibbets, Julie Pedersen, and Donna Gordon, who gave time out of their lives to be of service. And thank you to all those who sent cards and letters, and especially prayers, for my recovery. I will be forever grateful.

And, always to my husband Tom and our two dogs, Blaze and Lucky, who complete my life and bring me joy every day, who have shown me what it means to dance on life.

Introduction

The days drag by, every hour a struggle. But it's the nights I dread most. Exhausted, I lie in my bed, but sleep won't come. My friend is gone—the friend who got me through all the bad times, who was there for me whenever I needed help. Tears run down the sides of my face. Great sobs rack my body. How am I supposed to stop thinking about what happened—all that happened? Will I survive this without the help of my friend?

I've never known this much pain for so long—even when my kids died, or when my mother shot herself. Those times, of course, my friend was there to ease the pain, to help me sleep…or at least pass out. Is this grief? Can I really be grieving a bottle of whiskey? That's what a woman at a recovery meeting once told me. She said that I would grieve the loss of the one thing that could dull the feelings of guilt, shame, and disgust; and that all my unresolved grief would come to the surface, and it would have to be dealt with. Was she right?

All these years later, I'm in my own recovery from my addictions and working to help others. And something that same woman said to me dwells in the back of my mind. She said, "Even if you can stay in recovery from your addictions, as long as you hold on to the fear, anger, and grief, there's a good chance you'll either pick up another addiction, or return to a previous one." I've found that to be painfully true—in my life and in the lives of others.

Grief isn't solely about the death of a loved one. It's about loss.

Grief is great sorrow over loss, and *how much* sorrow we feel depends on how important something or someone was to us. Yes, I said "something." Grief isn't solely about the death of a loved one. It's about loss. We only die once in this lifetime, but we will suffer many losses along the way.

Consider the children who are victims of emotional, physical, and sexual abuse. They will grieve for their lost innocence. Rape victims grieve for the feelings of security and personal power that have been violently ripped from them. What about people who lose a part of their body, or suffer severe limitations due to a health problem? They will grieve for lost limbs, limited mobility, or the loss of freedom to do things their formerly sound body was able to do with ease. The list goes on.

There are those who are so invested in their careers or possessions that when those things are lost, it's as devastating as the death of a person might be. What about those people we lose not to death, but through a choice over which we have no control, like divorce? Sometimes it is more difficult to resolve grief when the person is still out in the world, walking around and having a life, while we dwell in sorrow.

There are two avenues one might travel when dealing with grief. One could feel it, deal with it, and struggle through the stages of grief to the point of acceptance. Alternately, one could move on with life, pushing the true feelings of grief down, ever fearful of experiencing them. People who follow this second avenue believe that having those feelings will surely kill them, and they will do whatever they can to avoid them.

One kind of denial is saying, "Nope. Didn't happen. Never." But denial is not really about denying what happened—it's about avoiding how you *feel* about the situation. And believe me when I tell you that grief will have its way, showing itself in your attitude and actions and weaseling its way into your relationships, until it is dealt with.

One of grief's favorite ways to show itself is through addictions. We don't consciously set out to be addicts. Addiction kind of sneaks up on us: a couple of drinks in the evening to relax; some pills to take the edge off; an evening of gambling as an escape; sexual release to blot out those undesirable feelings about ourselves; comfort food like mother used to make. Or we exhaust ourselves through overwork or cleaning; distract ourselves by shopping or using electronic devices; replace the pain by cutting and purging. The sad thing is that these things work for a while, dulling the grief, keeping our minds busy with other things, allowing us to forget about the problems, alleviating our need to be concerned about solutions...that is, until they become part of the problem.

Looking back, I understand that my grief began almost from the time I entered the world. I had an emotionally unavailable mother and an unhappy father who had his needs met at the expense of others. From a very young age I experienced every loss as a compounding of the grief that lived in me as fear and anger and which I later expressed with one addiction after another. My addiction became a merry-go-round that I couldn't get off of. I needed the addiction to deal with the pain, but I needed to hold on to the pain to justify the addiction.

Are you grieving? When did it begin? Are you stuck with guilt, denial, anger, depression, or self-destructive behavior? How are you acting out your grief? Do you know what it feels like to not be able to get off that merry-go-round?

If peace, happiness, and success seem impossible in your life, perhaps it's time to explore the *connection* between grief and addiction. Like the lady in the recovery meeting said, even if you remove the addictions from your life, if you hold on to the grief and continue to live in fear and anger, there's a good chance you will pick up a new addiction or continue to return to the previous one. Even if you don't, you'll live your life embittered by grief. To truly find relief is to walk through the grief process, confronting your fear and anger head on.

I know this to be true because I have trudged my way not only through addictions but through grief, and I've seen others do it, too. We've supported each other along the way, healed old wounds, released the burdens of our grief, and opened ourselves to all the possibilities this life has to offer. If you know, deep down in the most honest part of yourself, that you are suffering from grief and acting out through addictions, and you're seeking a way off that merry-go-round, come with me on a journey of discovery that will change your life forever. In this book, I will teach you what it means to dance on life.

Grieve It Forward

Most people have heard of the "pay it forward" concept: A person with no expectations commits a random act of kindness, the receiver of that kindness does the same for another, and on and on it goes. For those addicts holding fast to their grief, there is a similar concept I call "grieve it forward." A person with an agenda commits a specific act of cruelty to another, who then carries that into his or her day, and passes it on to another, and on and on it goes.

As kindnesses are paid forward, they tend to grow. And they also tend to come back to us. If we are kind to others, somehow it happens that others are kind to us. Or maybe it's just that we notice kindnesses.

Unfortunately the same is true with grief. When we treat someone cruelly—yell at a clerk or flip off another driver or some more serious breach—we not only hurt that person. We pretty much guarantee, unless they or someone else steps in to break the cycle, that the insult will be passed along. The world will be a bit meaner. And unless we can find a way to break the cycle of grieving forward, it's going to come back to us. Things are going to escalate. Even if it's only our own self we're nasty to, the principle still applies.

Years ago, I knew a woman who lived the "grieve it forward" concept to its fullest. Around the bars where she worked, others had nicknamed her "Smiley." Looking back, the irony isn't lost on me. Behind that perfect white smile—which, by the way, was as fake as she was—lived a pissed off woman who always had an agenda, and it certainly wasn't to help others or make their lives better.

Grieving for her early loss of innocence, any power and control she had over her life taken from her through rape, and feeling conflicted about what she thought life should be versus what she'd experienced, she lived mired in self-pity from a very young age. One by one, those closest to her hurt her, walked away, or died, and she turned to one addiction after another. She raged on this way for years, visiting her grief on everyone who crossed her path—she was grieving it forward in a major way.

I watched helplessly as she purposefully committed hateful, hurtful acts on others. It was as if releasing her fear and anger on another person would lessen her own pain. Instead, this cruelty merely compounded the feelings of guilt and shame she was trying so desperately to escape. I heard her blame everyone—including a God, who she professed didn't exist—and everything in her life, as she spiraled completely out of control and into the deep end of addiction, unable to get past denying her true feelings and anger.

I wanted to help, but the situation seemed hopeless. She would probably die like she'd lived—stuck in the early stages of grief. It would take a bigger person than I to help her find the way out of this downward spiral. I'd seen what had happened to those people who tried to help her: they either got dragged down with her, or she fought back so hard that they gave up for fear of going down with the ship.

You might be wondering who this woman was, what happened to her, how did I know her so intimately? She wasn't my mother, my sister, or a friend. Sadly, I must admit that she was me. During those years, it seemed like my life had split in two: the watcher and the actor. The watcher dwelled in shock and denial while the actor lived in pure anger, with many addictions.

Addicts will understand the concept of watcher and actor. It begins with the inability to move through the process of grief, and ends with the product—a behavior used to cope with a problem by becoming the problem. That's when the split happens. A part of the addict stands helplessly by, stunned, shocked, even appalled by his or her own actions, but fearful that to let go of the addiction would bring on a flood of unbearable emotions.

And they aren't necessarily wrong—except about the unbearable part.

If you had a 200-pound log to move, and someone offered to help you, wouldn't it just make sense to let the person help you carry the burden? That is the point of support groups, no matter whether you choose a church group, a grief group, or an addiction recovery program like the one I joined. The point is to make your burden bearable by allowing others to help you carry the load.

When I became tired of hopelessly standing by as the actor part of me raged on, committing unthinkable acts against myself and others, I sought out a 12-step meeting for alcoholics. I discovered that others in the group had joined

> If you had a 200-pound log to move, and someone offered to help you, wouldn't it just make sense to let the person help you carry the burden?

for the same reasons. Some of them had actually succeeded in finding their way not only to recovery from addiction, but to a place of peace, even happiness. Desperation may have driven me to the meeting, but curiosity kept me coming back. If it was possible for them, maybe there was hope for me too.

During my early years in recovery, I figured out that the "watcher, actor" concept could work in my favor if I applied it in a different way. Have you ever had one of those dreams where you are hovering around at a distance, watching yourself involved in some activity? It's like removing yourself from the situation. As part of my recovery program, it was necessary for me to look back over my life—what had been done to me, how I'd reacted. Through that process, I came face to face with the years of fear, anger, and grief that brought me to my addictions.

How did it happen? I stepped back, hovered nearby, and imagined the scenes from my life as if I were in a dream. Let me tell you, it was easier in my dreams! As I sat down with pen and paper to write out my inventory, I allowed the memories to return. That old familiar rage, self-pity for all the great sorrow I'd experienced, and fear of becoming overwhelmed grabbed my heart and twisted it. Bile began to rise. How in the world was I going to revisit the past without my old friend, whiskey, by my side?

It seemed like I'd left something out. Yes, I'd admitted my powerlessness over my addictions. I'd acknowledged that the power of "we" (the support group) could help me find some sanity in my otherwise insane thinking. But I hadn't yet been willing to open myself to the concept of a Higher Power. I was informed that until I could do that, my clever idea of using the "watcher, actor" concept in my recovery simply wouldn't work. Just as whiskey, drugs, and sex stood by me through the bad times, I would need a presence to hold my hand, to give me assurance as I relived those same situations. Although I didn't believe it at the time, I was told that my answers would come through complete surrender to a Higher Power of my choice. Oh my God! That was never going to happen!

Stuck, that helpless, hopeless watcher saw the actor continue on in her selfish, hateful, self-destructive ways, still visiting her grief on those around her. I wasn't using alcohol, drugs, or inappropriate sex anymore, but I thought about those things all day every day. I lived with a huge amount of resentment because I could no longer indulge in my addictions, and I spewed my venom around at every opportunity. I saw people at those meetings who had what I wanted, who gave me hope. Believe me, I'm sure no new-comer encountered me and thought, "That's what I want."

As stuck as I was, fighting the urges every day, struggling with the strange thoughts that constantly flitted through my mind, and fear-ing moving forward into the unknown, there was still a part of me that didn't want to go back to the life I'd known before. What if I did it—surrendered to some Higher Power—and I didn't like his plan for me? My anger said, "Every time you prayed before, it turned out bad." My fear said, "What if it doesn't work for you? What if you put it all out there and fail? What if this God doesn't think you deserve happiness?" But then my misery whispered loudest, "If you're planning on sticking around, you'd better do something. Nothing else you've tried has worked. Why not give it a shot?"

Have you experienced the split into watcher and actor? What is your watcher seeing? Is your actor doing things that go against your true nature? Have you jumped on the grief/addiction merry-go-round and can't seem to get off? Are you grieving it forward, hurting the people you profess to care about, denying yourself the very things you say you want?

The solution is simple, but not easy. The good news is that you are not alone, unless you choose to be. There are many of us out there who have gone through the same things you're experiencing. We've found a way out, and we are willing to share that with you. Your job in this scenario is to acknowledge your problem, ask for help, and be willing to do whatever it takes to find recovery not only from your addiction, but from fear, anger, and grief.

Living Proof

A commonly held concept of faith is that it is believing in something for which there is no "proof." But what is proof but determining a certainty based on results? Imagine a person whose life had been consumed with thoughts of drinking, drugging, and dying, who, through a sincere act of faith, began the journey to a life beyond her capabilities alone.

All I wanted was some peace, to be able to shut the dark thoughts from my mind, to sleep through the night without fear of waking in terror. I wanted to function without having to drink myself into oblivion. To wake up in the morning without that feeling of dread brought on by my grief over all I'd lost—without the need to constantly feed my addictions—would have been enough. But I received so much more.

I could share with you how I arrived at that moment when I fell to my knees, surrendered, and asked for help. But I think it's more important to tell you the results of my first encounter with a Higher Power. My discovery wasn't like a magic wand that changed my circumstances, but it was the beginning of seeing things through new eyes. As soon as I took the action and said the words, "I give up. I need help," something grabbed the other end of that 200-pound log that I'd been trying to move alone for thirty-five years, and I knew I could move forward.

As I repeated the same thing each morning, subtle changes took place. I felt like someone had taken my hand and was showing me the way to go—I felt safe and loved for the first time in a long time. No longer did I live with that feeling of being a rudderless ship in a raging ocean. I'd seen the star that would lead me to solid ground, and a better way to live. I can't recall ever knowing that feeling in my life before I found my Higher Power. It was better than getting high.

My discovery of my Higher Power wasn't like a magic wand that changed my circumstances, but it was the beginning of seeing things through new eyes.

As time passed I noticed that I was looking at others differently. Before, I'd always resented those who had more than me. I was filled with envy and bitterness for anyone who I believed hadn't suffered as much as I had. After I found my Higher Power, I began seeing these people clearly—hearing them with my heart instead of my ears. Their pain was as real to them as mine was to me, and comparing pain was like comparing apples and oranges.

This profound change became clear to me one night when I went to a speaker meeting in the small town where I lived at the time. It was one of those little towns where everyone thinks they know everything about the other residents, and I was acquainted with the man who would be sharing his recovery story. I can remember wondering how he fell into addiction, what he was doing in a 12-step meeting. He had everything: money, cars, property, a family, and the choice to live his life any way he wanted... all the things I thought I needed to be happy, so why wasn't he? Early on I figured he was stupid, that he didn't deserve all that he had. But that night I was curious, and I stuck around to hear his story.

As I listened to the man speak, I was filled with unfamiliar emotions. Tears rolled down my face. This man may have had more than I, but we weren't so different. He'd grown up with a demanding, controlling father who expected total compliance and excellence in everything he did. And no matter how hard he tried and how well he did, it was never good enough, which translated to him that *he* wasn't good enough. The only port in his otherwise tense life was his mother, who, like my mother, took her own life. He'd spent his life achieving and accumulating things, but he lived in fear of never being good enough, choked with anger toward his father, who'd ruined his childhood, and his mother, who'd deserted him when he needed her most. He was grieving for the little boy who'd been denied the love and acceptance all of us want.

I couldn't believe I was weeping for this wealthy businessman who was looked up to in our small town. There was a time before my spiritual connection when I would have thought things like: "What a whiner. He needs to get over himself. He's got it all. His kids are alive, he doesn't have to struggle for every penny. My life is so much worse than his. What is his problem?" But that night I understood that although our lives had been different in many ways, inside each of us lived the same hurt, frightened, angry child, stuck in grief and seeking escape through addiction.

As I was sitting in the local coffee shop one morning, I heard the news: this man was dead. He'd taken his own life. I'd gotten to know him over the past year, and I understood his struggle with spirituality and the idea of surrender. He'd relapsed several times, but he always returned to the meetings, sad and sorry, but unable or unwilling to find faith. Through his death, I learned to have compassion for myself. I only wish he could have seen himself through my eyes. He had a good heart, was kind and compassionate. But he couldn't give himself what he needed most, and he refused to ask for spiritual help. He carried his burden alone until the weight of it was too much.

Like my friend, I sometimes struggled with the spiritual connection, but instead of stepping backwards, I fell to my knees and begged for help until the doubts passed. What I discovered was that finding faith isn't a onetime thing. Each day is a new beginning, with new opportunities and different circumstances, and if I'm to navigate, I need a God of my understanding to lead the way. There may be times when I'm not certain of what to do, but there is never a time when I don't know what *not* to do.

I can share with you how I found faith. Others can do the same. You can read books; listen to speakers; attend support groups, therapy, or church. But finding faith is as unique as each individual, and it is a very personal experience. It's not "thinking" that there is a Higher Power— it's *knowing* it with unfaltering certainty. If you are looking for proof of a Higher Power, of how faith can change a life, the only way you'll find it is within yourself.

What happened to that 200-pound log I'd been carrying around? A God of my understanding began carrying half the burden, and as I moved through the twelve steps, I whittled down those feelings of fear, anger, and grief little by little until I was free of it altogether. Without help, without divine intervention, I could not have done it. That is proof enough for me.

Keep in mind that sometimes you have to get down before you can stand up.

The Storm Within

Brace yourself! A storm is building. The flood will come. For as long you've been active in your addiction, you've been building a protective wall to keep your emotions at bay. Once you're in recovery, the wall will begin to crumble, and soon you'll be flooded with emotions. Just as you had to hit a life bottom with your addiction, sooner or later you will hit an emotional bottom with your fear, anger, and grief.

I'm reminded of a story I heard years ago. A flood swept over the countryside. As the water rose, a man climbed higher and higher in his house until he stood on the roof. He wasn't worried, because he knew that God would save him. When a rescue boat came by, he waved it away, saying, "God will save me." Meanwhile, the water kept rising. A helicopter flew overhead. He waved it away, saying, "God will save me." The house tumbled into the raging water, and the man died. When he awoke in Heaven, he said to God, "I thought you were going to save me." God said, "I sent you a boat and a helicopter. What more did you want?"

The boat is other people in the same circumstances who can help you, and the helicopter is a Higher Power sending you a lifeline. Unless you are willing to get in the boat or grab the lifeline, you will be lost in the flood. The moral of the story is that unless you are willing to accept help, you will be left standing atop a flooded house with nothing to grab hold of.

> Unless you are willing to accept help, you will be left standing atop a flooded house with nothing to grab hold of.

Over the course of my years in recovery, I've seen many go it alone: they slip under the water and then struggle to the surface, rebuilding their great wall as they struggle to manage their on-again/off-again addiction cycle.

There are others who do not return to their addictions, but refuse to take down that protective wall. I recall the story of one woman, who had over twenty years of sobriety but showed up at every meeting in crisis and tears. At that time, I didn't understand. But today I do. She was sober, but the storm within raged on.

How will you know when you are going to hit your emotional bottom? It's different for everyone, but there are signs. Like many others, when I entered a recovery program, I walked through the doors of a 12-step meeting with attitude, wearing the facade that I'd lived through so much crap that no one could hurt me. Looking back, I was quite the macho broad, and I didn't trust anyone. Trust is a big issue with addicts. We protect our vulnerable side by wearing one mask or another. It takes time to rip those masks away and allow others to see us as we really are—especially when we've been unable to trust others for so many years.

Years ago, while working as a costume designer, I had the privilege of making costumes for professional clowns. Ignorant about the profession, I wrongly assumed that these people threw on a colorful costume, painted their faces, and acted funny. I was so wrong! It takes an incredible amount of work to develop an alternate persona. Isn't that exactly what we addicts do?

As I spent time working on their costumes, I thought of all I'd learned about the clowns. I wondered, what costume, face, and personality did I wear while active in my addictions? In my imagination, my addict personality was named "Jiggles," and she was dressed in sexy clown clothes that accentuated her ample chest and narrow hips. She had lines painted above and below her eyes, and severely arched eyebrows to indicate her toughness. Oversized glasses showed how smart she was, and a big red smile said that she was okay. Finally, she had one tiny little tear at the corner of each eye—so small you barely noticed them.

"Jiggles" would sashay around the ring, shyly peeking out from behind a ruffled umbrella. When you got too close to her, the umbrella would transform into a squirt gun, and she'd shoot you in the face and run away. The difference between me and the clowns I made costumes for was that at the end of their work day, the clowns removed their make-up and clothes and returned to real life. I lived in my fantasy.

The first sign that something was about to happen—that a storm was brewing inside me—was when those tiny tears became real tears. After my initial struggle with recovery, as I settled into going to meetings, living differently, finding hope, and having the burden of addiction removed, I went through a euphoric period. I was over two years clean, sober, and not acting out sexually. I felt uncharacteristically emotional. I started crying at the slightest provocation—a sad story, a television show, or a certain song on the radio was enough to make unbidden tears start gushing from my eyes. At first I thought I was losing my mind. I wasn't one of those criers I judged harshly in the meetings. Why couldn't I control the tears?

When the tears come of their own volition, triggered by waves of emotions set off by one trigger or another, it's time to grab that lifeline, because you are in for a bumpy ride. You are about to be swamped by the feelings of grief that you've kept at bay through your addiction or addictive behavior. Your emotional bottom is at hand. This is the point when true recovery—not only from addiction, but from the storm within—begins.

The "G" List

When you hit your emotional bottom, you've reached the point in recovery that separates the willing from the unwilling. This is when you must take action toward your goal. Where do you begin?

Begin at the beginning. The "G" (grief) list will help you understand where, when, and how fear, anger, and grief took control of your life. First, find a quiet place. Sit comfortably, close your eyes, and try to picture the last time in your life when you felt reasonably safe, happy, and content. I don't mean a fleeting moment of happiness, but a time when you knew real *contentment*. When you have it clearly in your mind, stop and write it down.

When was it?

Where were you?

Who was there?

What was happening?

When faced with this exercise, I wrote:

When: 1953

Where: Kaskaskia River, just outside Cowden, Illinois

Who: My grandfather, his wife, my brother, me, and our dog, Pedro

What: Spending the summer before I started school at the river with Grampa. It was a glorious summer—we swam and played in the river, fished, hunted, made pies from berries we picked, ate corn from the field, and helped Grampa make doughballs for the trout lines placed along the banks of the river. Grampa traded for an old row boat, fixed it up, painted my name on the side, and gave it to me for my sixth birthday.

Next, go back to that time and consider what changed that altered how you felt.

Was it something that happened to you?

Was it something you did?

Who was there?

What were the circumstances?

Stop and write it down. This will be the beginning of your "G" (grief) list.

I wrote:

When: 1953, last day at the river

Where: In the car on the way back to town

Who: My mom, my dad, my brother, me, and the dog

What: Tension between Mom and Dad in the car. Mom popped the top on a beer and kept looking over the back of her seat, glaring at me and talking about school starting in a week. She insisted that there was much to be done to get me ready. I wouldn't be able to run around like a heathen, looking like something the cat dragged in anymore. Something would have to be done with my stringy hair. She'd been given some secondhand dresses that would work, but we would have to buy some new shoes.

I could feel a tightening in my belly as I looked down at myself. Tears threatened to spill over, but I pushed them back. Crying was not acceptable, even when I got a whipping. I wanted to jump from the car, run back to the river, and never go back to town.

The following week changed my life, and not for the better. My river-tanned dark skin and the home permanent that left me with a burnt, bushy blob of hair surrounding my face didn't help matters. Fear gripped my heart as I entered the huge brick building in my ill-fitting dress and too-tight shoes.

My fear was not unfounded. I didn't look like the other girls. Kids made fun of my dark skin, calling me names I didn't understand. I wanted to run away, to hide, but there was no place to go. I shoved the fear and hurt deep down inside, and allowed those feelings to be replaced by anger. I lashed out at every opportunity. I couldn't focus on school, because I was locked in a fight to survive day by day—or so it felt. My teachers and classmates thought that I was stupid.

This was the person I carried into the next twenty-nine years of my life: the person who grabbed on to one addiction after another to conceal the fear, anger, and grief that lived inside her; the person who, when other losses occurred, piled them on top of the old feelings until the burden eventually became that unmovable 200-pound log.

Once you've discovered the beginning of your "G" list, you can go on to discover how you piled on additional feelings of fear, anger, and grief. What you get out of this list is clarity— about where it all started, why, how you reacted, and how you've incorporated old feelings into the life you live today. You can't find a solution to a problem until you understand the problem.

Why is it important to write this all down? Getting it out of you is cathartic, and it shows a willingness to put thoughts of recovery into action. Things look different in black and white...more real. If you think you can do this as a mental exercise, you will likely get distracted and stop thinking about it. Writing it down is about actually making a real, tangible commitment to your own recovery. What you get out of it depends on what you are willing to put in.

If you continue to write out the experiences that have shaped your life and brought you to your addiction with brutal honesty, you will not only relive memories, but feel things that you've attempted to escape for years. That's why it's important to have a support system in place. This is a very vulnerable time—a time when friends and your connection to a Higher Power might be the only lifelines that can keep you from stepping backward, from seeking those old escapes and distractions. For me, it was very important to have people who understood because they'd been through the same problems. It is wonderful to have a supportive family, friends, a minister, and others, but if they have not faced what you're facing, even if they have the best of intentions, they

> You can't find a solution to a problem until you understand the problem.

can't truly understand. That can cause frustration for all involved.

This is not an *easy* solution, but it is the beginning of a *real* solution to those questions in your mind through which all other thoughts and decisions are filtered, i.e.: What's wrong with me? Why do I do the things I do? Why can't I stop? Am I stupid, or just crazy? Why does it seem like everyone else can figure things out, and I can't? Is there no hope for me?

There is hope, if you are willing to go back and re-experience feeling what you were feeling when you were feeling it, and commit it to paper. Until you can do that, those suppressed emotions and questions in your mind will be your burden to carry, and they will influence every decision you make and every relationship you have from that moment on.

As a result of writing out my "G" list, which was quite extensive, I achieved a clearer understanding of myself and the people important to me. I discovered that I was not evil, bad, crazy, stupid, or hopeless, but I had made a lot of poor choices based on fear, anger, and grief. My parents, in treating me poorly when I was growing up, were reacting to their own fear, anger, and grief. It wasn't about me—it was about them, and the addictions they used to escape their true feelings. Teachers and others who knew nothing of what was going on with me (because I refused to acknowledge it) were reacting to my behavior, which was completely out of control. I couldn't expect anyone to understand how I was feeling until I found a way to put it into words. After considering my past, and the root of my addictions, I was able to put my regrets aside and welcome a new day, filled with fresh awareness and the opportunity to make healthier choices.

Unexpressed feelings don't merely disappear. They go somewhere inside you, into a dark place where resentments hide and fester. If you don't think they influence you in every facet of your life, you are fooling yourself. Until you become willing to take each one out, feel it, and express it in a healthy way, it will be a guiding force in your life.

> Unexpressed feelings don't merely disappear. They go somewhere inside you, into a dark place where resentments hide and fester.

Doing the "G" list is the beginning of taking positive action toward your recovery. Having raged through life for so many years, it seemed like a monumental task for me.

However, my 12-step program had taught me to break things down into smaller bites. Therefore, I only bit off what I could process at one time, which gave me ample space to get through all of it. As painful as it was, I know that I would do it all over again for the feeling I found on the other side.

If you have trouble sorting it all out and figuring out what is still affecting your life, and why, look for the clues that are right in front of you. These clues will become apparent when you have experiences that trigger emotional responses in you. Even though you may have become proficient at suppressing emotions by running back to your addiction for solace, the feelings were real, and they came from somewhere in your life.

Do you have fears associated with having real intimacy and trusting another human being? Why? When did it begin? Who was the prominent person in your life who hurt and disappointed you? For instance, because I never experienced a bond with my mother and believed she didn't like me, for the first half of my life I had no women friends. I had no concept of how to relate to other women. Grieving for my mother's love, I carried that fear of being hurt into relationships and kept potential female friends at an arm's length, waiting for the other shoe to drop. During those years, when I'd watch a movie or television show about women who truly cared for each other, tears of sorrow would well up from the deepest part of me, sending me reeling toward one of my addictions.

Do you find yourself reacting with anger in situations that most people would tolerate? The truth is that anger is a cop-out for those who refuse to deal with their real emotions. Imagine a person who is unhappy in his life, frustrated because it hasn't turned out the way he'd expected. He gets in his car and at the smallest infraction from another driver, reacts with road rage. All the rage from this man's past is triggered just by someone pulling out in front of him. And because he never got to share his true feelings with whomever actually hurt him in the past, he takes it out on a complete stranger.

If you're wondering how to start your grief list, consider those things that trigger deep-seated feelings, and how you react to them. What situations in movies, television shows, or real life bring on tears of sorrow that you might convert into a feeling of self-pity or anger? How do you use anger to disguise other feelings that make you uncomfortable? Are you using addiction in an attempt to distract yourself from the truth? It may work temporarily, but your grief will live on until you take it out, dust it off, and acknowledge how it has affected the way you live and react to the world around you. The "G" list can take you to a place of understanding that can not only help you in recovery from your addictions, but also from fear, anger, and grief.

Whispers and Screams

Ready or not, it will happen: the day when a person is expected to transform from a child into an adult, when it is time to put away childish things. What are childish things? Children, as is natural, are totally self-involved, and they do whatever it takes to get their needs met. They will do everything from people-pleasing to throwing tantrums to get what they want.

It's been said that the point in a person's life when they become addicted is the point they will stay at emotionally until the addiction is addressed. People who had a hard time with the transition from childhood to adulthood will be stuck as self-involved children, running around in big bodies with stunted brains, trying to make adult decisions. If you think the chaos around these people is bad, think about what it must be like to live in their heads.

I'm reminded of that scene that's in movies, cartoons, even commercials, where the main characters are faced with a decision, and they have help. On one shoulder they have an angel and on the other, a devil. Both are trying to convince them of what to do. If I ever had an angel attempting to tell me the right thing to do, it was many years ago, and as soon as I became addicted, she got knocked off by another devil. On one shoulder the devil, who represented fear and grief, whispered in my ear—and on the other, anger and addiction screamed at me.

Fear and grief reminded me constantly of all I missed out on in life, and all that I lost. A devil crouched on one shoulder, whispering in my ear, saying things like: "Go ahead and have another drink. Take that pill—you deserve it after all you've been through. It's okay to get involved with him, so what if he's married? It's not your problem. Just make sure you don't get too close so when it ends, you won't get hurt. No one understands your pain. No one really loves you. They deserve what they get. You're only doing what you have to, to survive."

On the other shoulder, the red-faced, stomping little devil raged on, screaming about how unfair my life had been, reminding me what shoulda, coulda, woulda been, if only my life had been different. I would share with you the words, but that little devil had a really filthy mouth. At that time, I might be smiling at your face, making the right noises to get what I wanted, but the words in my mind didn't match what I said out loud.

Like a child who blames his sibling, pet, friends, or parents for the bad things he does, I blamed other people and situations for my behavior. I even convinced myself that I was justified in my actions, which was handy because it got me off the hook and allowed me the perfect excuse to continue living the way I lived.

It all began with grief. As a child, I grieved for the life I thought I should have had, for the people I wanted my parents to be, for the person I wanted to be but wasn't—and with each new disappointment and betrayal, my grief turned to fear that I expressed with anger and tried to escape through addictions.

That is the person I carried into early recovery from my addictions. It wasn't pretty. My devils rode with me everywhere I went, making my life a living hell. Even as I sat in 12-step meetings, listening to the stories of others who'd found recovery, my little devils continued to whisper and scream the phrases that would surely take me back to my addictions. The fact that I'd had to give up the only things that numbed my grief and distracted me from reality only made things worse. My fear devil would whisper, "You're not that bad, all things considered. You shouldn't have to give up the only things that get you through the day, that take the pain away. What's going to happen if you try this and it doesn't work? What will you do then? Are you hopeless?" Then my anger devil would scream profanities in my ear, telling me, "These people are full of crap. They don't know you. They haven't had to live your life, to deal with all you've been through. Who the hell do they think they are to tell you how to live your life?"

One thing I discovered was that it wasn't going to get better until I became willing to put in some effort. Babies take baby steps, and God knows I was one big baby.

I'm not sure what kept me going back to those meetings, but I did. Maybe it was because, underneath it all, I knew the truth. Maybe it was because no matter how badly I acted, the people there treated me well and kept telling me that things would get better. One thing I discovered was that it wasn't going to get better until I became willing to put in some effort.

Babies take baby steps, and God knows I was one big baby. I was still lying, manipulating, and blaming, and I had to find a way to stop.

As I began to trust other people in the meetings, I found myself attempting to make a connection to a Higher Power. I would lie in my bed night after night, unable to sleep, listening to the whispers and screams. A woman told me that I would not know relief until I wrote out my grief list. Then she said, "But that is only the beginning. There will come a time when it will be necessary for you to say it out loud to a God of your understanding and another human being."

I remember my fear devil speaking up at that time to inform me that I couldn't do that. First of all, who would I tell? If I did find someone to tell, what would they think of me if they knew the whole truth? And of course, my anger devil broke in to add that telling another person about my wrongs was stupid. What difference would it make? If there was a God, he already knew everything anyway. They couldn't make me do it.

But then something else happened. A third voice, a new voice, spoke up and said, "Why not give it a try? It seems to have worked for others. What's the worst thing that could happen if you let it all out?"

I listened to the new voice. My grief list in hand, I sought out a person I trusted and told him everything. I was amazed that he didn't scorn me, tell me what a bad person I was, or turn and walk away in disgust. He simply told me, as others had, that things would get better. It would take time, but they would get better. I slept soundly that night for the first time in a long time. It was all out there now, all my dirty little secrets, and the world hadn't come to an end.

Do you know what it is to hear the devils whispering in your ears? The only way to rid yourself of your fears is to give yourself a voice. Before recovery, when I heard that confession was good for the soul, I didn't understand. But I do now. There is something about putting it all out there that takes all the power away from the whispers and screams. Releasing secrets that you may have carried for years, and knowing that they can never come back to hurt you again, brings a permanent relief unlike anything addiction ever could.

Will it be difficult and painful? Yes, it will. But there are times when pain can be a good thing.

Through pain, our bodies tell us there is something wrong. That hit home for me once when I was speaking to a woman who had been abusing painkillers for years. She said, "Hell, I keep myself so numb, I wouldn't know it if I had some horrible disease that was going to kill me." I thought that the same applies to our emotional pain. It's there to get our attention, to tell us what needs to be done.

When it was time for me, I paced back and forth in the kitchen of a trusted friend, openly weeping, as I shared the story of my life. I cried out how I'd blamed my father for every failed relationship with men I'd ever had. He hurt me. He left me. He got another family. The pain I felt every time I saw him with them was nearly unbearable. I hated him and I took it out on other men. I never gave myself fully because I didn't want to experience the pain of loss when the man betrayed me, and I was convinced all of them would.

The realization I came to through reliving the pain around my father was how unfair I'd been. My childlike mind took the whole thing personally. When I heard the words come out of my mouth, it dawned on me that my father was in pain. He'd become an alcoholic, but he didn't leave *me*—he left an unbearable situation in which my mom was having an affair with his brother. As each of my grievances found their way into words, as I wept over my losses, one thing kept coming to the surface: empathy. I learned the ability to empathize with others. In the past, I hadn't been able to get past my own pain to see that *others* were in pain, too—and were doing what they felt they had to do to survive.

As difficult as it was to tell it all, to take responsibility for my part in situations and relationships, there came an understanding and some relief in speaking the truth. I was finally *feeling* the feelings I'd avoided for so many years. From the age of eight, when I first stole one of my mother's tranquilizers, to the years of drinking, other drugs, and acting out sexually, I'd dealt with my fear, anger, and grief through addictions. Beneath the surface, the pain festered and continued to affect my life. There was not enough alcohol, drugs, or anything else that could wipe out my feelings. The only thing that worked was putting them into words, and acknowledging the truth. No matter how old I was, up to that point, I'd lived my life as an emotionally stunted eight-year-old.

Consider how old you were when you began to use an addiction to suppress your feelings, when the devils climbed on your shoulders to whisper self-pitying justifications into one ear, and scream obscenities at others into the other. Be brutally honest, because it's not about anyone but you. Say the words, allow yourself to feel what you were truly feeling at the time, and finally let it go. Is this the only solution? I don't know, but I do know it was the only solution that worked for me.

Excuse Me? I'm Addicted

Picture this: A fancy hotel dining room with white linen tablecloths, shiny stemware, sparkling glasses, and a beautiful centerpiece on each table. I was sitting in such a room with four others I knew from recovery meetings, anticipating a wonderful lunch before we went to one of the huge meeting rooms to hear a very special speaker. The young waiter approached, filled our glasses with water, and said, "May I get you something from the bar?"

"We are trying not to drink," a man with over twenty years in recovery snapped at him. The waiter stood in stunned silence, unsure how to respond. I could have crawled under the table. Finally, the waiter turned and said, "Well, isn't that special," and walked away. My tablemate was livid and wouldn't let it go. He stormed from the table to speak to the manager. I don't know what happened to the waiter, but I never saw him again.

Lunch was a tense affair, the rest of us embarrassed by the man's actions but saying nothing. I don't know if we were intimidated by the man's long-term sobriety or afraid that he would turn his wrath upon us. I could feel my anger building, the screaming in my head yelling at me to do something. Instead, I continued to put food in my mouth that by that time tasted like cardboard.

It wasn't until we were in the car on the way home that I decided I couldn't keep my mouth shut any longer. As the man, who was driving, raged on about the incident, I said, "What is wrong with you? It's not like we were sitting in wheelchairs with signs around our necks proclaiming we were alcoholics." My comment did no good as far as the man was concerned, but I certainly felt better for saying it.

It takes a lot of courage and effort to find real recovery not only from our addictions, but from those things that were in place that brought us to the addictions.

Alone, at home, I recalled something I'd heard around the meetings. Someone said, "You take a drunken jackass and sober him up, and all you have is a sober jackass." It takes a lot of courage and effort to find real recovery not only from our addictions, but from those things that brought us to the addictions. We are not special, except in our inability to handle those things most people handle all their lives, without seeking an easier, softer way. That's not something to take great pride in.

Addiction can be an explanation, but it is not an excuse. When we bring the same self-centered, angry, grieving person with us into recovery; when we are unwilling to look at who we were and make changes accordingly, what's the point? Person-

> Addiction can be an explanation, but it is not an excuse.

ally, I found that writing my grief list out—giving voice to all that had happened, what I'd done, who I'd become—was a humbling experience. I knew through this new awareness that there were no excuses left; it was time to learn to live like a decent human being.

Deep down, I think I always wanted to be decent, but until I became aware of the self-sabotaging things I did, it wasn't going to happen. The truth is that there was no one to blame but myself. I'd cheated myself out of wonderful experiences and healthy relationships— the very life I spent years whining that I wanted. I certainly wasn't special—I was simply a sad case.

The people around us might be able to see our character defects clearly, but until we see them and understand that they are a problem, they will continue to destroy our lives. I can only imagine some of the things that were said about me when

I walked out of a room. Others probably said things like: "She's a mess. What in the world is she thinking? Obviously, she's not thinking. I wonder what's going to happen to her? I don't know, but it probably won't be good." And those are some of the nicer things I can imagine!

How do you suppose others see you? What might they say about you when you leave the room? Why do you think that is? Is there any truth to it? Are you the person you want to be, or the person you think you *have* to be because you are addicted? If you are the latter, you'll discover that it was never a viable excuse. Addiction may have been an explanation for your inappropriate behavior, but it does not excuse it.

Grieving addicts believe they are entitled to be the people they are, that others should put up with them because their life has been so tough, one way or another. Well, life is tough for most people. Life is a series of challenges, and if we are to face them in recovery, we must take a hard look at who we have been and why we felt it was okay to act out through addictions. We must be willing to do whatever it takes to live life on *life's* terms, like those non-addicted individuals. We say we never felt as if we fit in—well, this is the solution to fitting in with the rest of the world.

Convincing yourself that you are "special" because you suffer from addiction—and holding on to the attitude that others should cater to you, make allowances for you, or compromise themselves because of your problem—is a clear indication that although you may have set aside your addiction, you are still holding on to fear, anger, and grief. You might as well stick your hand in others' faces and say, "Excuse me? I'm addicted."

Authentic recovery isn't attitude—it's humility. Humility comes through the honest appraisal of your life, of the person you became while indulging in your addiction. Humility is about putting aside your fear and false pride to ask for help, and having gratitude for an opportunity to become the person you want to be.

Humility is about putting aside your fear and false pride to ask for help, and having gratitude for an opportunity to become the person you want to be.

Once, when faced with making the decision to complete a difficult task that would help in my recovery, I balked. I said to another person in the same recovery program, "I have my pride." To my surprise, the person responded by smiling and saying, "Where was your precious pride when you were falling off bar stools and screwing everyone in town?" That certainly put it into perspective for me. What about you? Where was your pride when you were indulging in your addiction, doing things you wouldn't dream of doing in recovery?

The wise check their attitude at the door as they step over the threshold to a new way of life. They understand that to be humble is not the same as humiliation. If they don't, they should, because I'm sure that they experienced humiliation while living as addicts. There is nothing humiliating about addressing a serious problem, asking for help, and accepting it. If you had cancer, you wouldn't hesitate to go to a doctor or ask for help, to do whatever it took to regain your quality of life. How different is this, really?

Strange Packages

After you've written out your grief list, come to an understanding of why you fell into addiction, and taken responsibility for your behavior, it's time to make a crucial decision. What are you going to do about it? Many addicts spend so much energy protecting and feeding their addiction that they become unrecognizable, even to themselves.

Changing old habits, especially ones that are bad for you, can be a difficult task. But if you are seeking real recovery, the kind that involves peace and serenity, it is essential. When I first heard that, I remember hating the thought of peace and serenity, saying to myself, "What a bore *that* would be." If I found peace and serenity, I would be like everyone else. I wouldn't be special anymore. Holding on to the drama created by those things was the only thing that made me feel different, special, and justified my addictions.

I recently heard a man say that when non-addicted people have a flat tire, they call for roadside assistance. When addicts have a flat tire, they call the suicide hotline. Addicts absolutely thrive on drama. As long as they hold on to whatever painful experiences and losses they've gone through, they can excuse their current behavior by pulling out that old stuff and using it to nail themselves to a cross for all the world to see.

The great martyr routine only works for a while before others get tired of it and start dropping out of our lives like rats from a sinking ship. Only extremely determined addicts can make that work for them—by convincing themselves that no one loves them, no one understands, which creates even more drama and excuses. It takes a lot of work and focus to continue creating drama. It may involve lying, cheating, making others look bad so you don't seem so bad in comparison, an inability to empathize with others for fear of losing the attention you crave, and total focus on self to the exclusion of those around you.

Of the things we hang on to that keep us from happier, healthier lives in recovery, two of the most common are the highs and lows created by making mountains of molehills, and total self-involvement. When you can find a way to change those things, many of your other shortcomings will fall by the wayside. After all, you will eliminate the need to lie about circumstances to make them seem more dramatic than they actually were. You won't have to talk badly about others to keep them from finding out the truth about you; you'll stop attempting to steal attention through extreme measures; and you'll be able to have real relationships that include the needs of other involved persons.

How do we let go of our shortcomings—the ones that we've used to skate through life, manipulating others and deluding ourselves for so long? It was suggested to me that I might ask this God of my understanding to help me. That seemed simple enough. What I didn't realize at the time was that my answers might come wrapped in strange packages.

I asked for patience, which was not my strong suit. It wasn't like this God waved his hand and put a spell on me, and suddenly I was filled with patience. No, that would be way too easy. He gave me opportunities to practice patience, such as: lines to stand in, oftentimes behind elderly people counting pennies from a coin purse; rude drivers who raced in front of me to take "my" parking space; phone calls from pushy telemarketers; people who wanted to share their problems

> It wasn't like this God waved his hand and put a spell on me, and suddenly I was filled with patience.

with me, many of which didn't seem nearly as bad as mine; and others in meetings who told me the truth whether I wanted to hear it or not.

Like the emotionally stunted child I was, I had to learn patience, and that required practicing it each day in so many situations. A dear friend once told me that we become what we practice; opportunities are put in front of us as chances to put into practice what we said we wanted.

As time passed and I stayed in recovery, I was given a tremendous number of opportunities, which apparently the God of my understanding knew I needed, until this new way of thinking became second nature. My anger turned to patience, fear to faith, grief to joy. I channeled my grief into the knowledge that it took everything in my life to bring me to the present moment—to being a person of value who had something to give back to others and the world around her.

There is an old adage that goes: "Be careful what you ask for; you just might get it." I think they should add, "...and you might be surprised *how* you get it." Like any other skill, these life lessons take time and practice. Since I didn't learn these things earlier in life, I had to learn them in my recovery. The main objective is to remain teachable and to pay attention to those opportunities. Yes, you can teach an old drunk new tricks.

Frenemies

Frenemies: a new word for a human condition that's been around since the beginning of the human race. I call these people the "what have you done for me lately" people. A true friend cares at least as much for his friend's feelings as his own. If you cannot function as a friend, there's not much hope for other relationships. The problem for addicts is that the addiction always looms between them and their friends.

In *Sand and Foam*, Kahlil Gibran said, "Friendship is a sweet responsibility, never an opportunity." Not so for me. While actively addicted, I looked at every relationship as an opportunity to work people, to get my needs met, no matter what it cost them. I acted like I was their friend, but in the back of my mind I wondered: What can I get out of this? How can this relationship benefit me?

If you cannot function as a friend, there's not much hope for other relationships.

I blamed my family for what a wreck my life was. I took what I could get from them and walked away without looking back. I used my son to fill my need for unconditional love, but was not capable of giving him the same. I changed friends, lovers, and husbands like most people change their seasonal wardrobe, depending on my needs at the time. When I was finished with them, when they had nothing left that I wanted, it was over for me—and I didn't understand why they were so upset with me. I'd moved on to another mark...what was their problem? They were so needy. That's the way my mind worked.

Before I started recovery, I didn't realize that it would be necessary for me to revisit the hurt I'd caused those who'd been unfortunate enough to cross my path. Looking back, I believe there were people who really cared for me, but I cast them aside like so much trash when they stopped or refused to fill my needs. I'm sure I was like a black hole, sucking up everything around me but never getting filled up. Then, one day, there was no one left—no one to blame, no one to love me, no one to use up. All that was left was me and my fear, anger, grief, and by then, many addictions.

Throughout my young life there were people who hurt me, who disappointed me, who didn't live up to my expectations. Unable or unwilling to deal with that pain, I grieved, but not in a healthy way.

I masked my fear of intimacy, of trusting others, with anger. Anger was the only emotion that made me feel as if I had any power at all. It was also the emotion I used to justify my addictions. I carried that anger into every interaction I had, and then wondered why all my relationships failed. In the back of my sick mind I believed that as long as I could get them before they got me, I could survive.

What I discovered in recovery was that life is about more than simply surviving. I'd made a mess of everything, and I had to clean it up if I hoped to know any peace. With pen and paper, I sat down and started a list of all those I'd harmed. I understood that it didn't matter what they did to me, but how I acted or reacted to the situation. There were relatives I'd been punishing for years. I withheld compassion and affection from them, and at every opportunity attempted to make them as miserable as I was. I made no attempt to understand the circumstances that made other people who they were, what drove them to do the things they did. Ironically, I expected everyone to understand and sympathize with me, but I was not willing to do that for them.

> What I discovered in recovery was that life is about more than simply surviving.

The last name I added to the list was my own. Looking back, I don't think anyone could have hurt me any worse than I hurt myself. Even though I constantly told myself that I had good reason to treat others badly, nurtured my anger, and held fast to my grief, there was a part of me that carried guilt and shame for my thoughts and actions. That was not the person I wanted to be, so I used my addictions to smother those feelings.

Think of all the people you've harmed in your life. Try writing their names down. If you put aside what you believe they did to hurt you, real or imagined, and focus on the ways you acted on that, what do you see? Have you carried those feelings into your life since then, and used them to punish yourself and new people who had nothing to do with what happened to you earlier on? Now, look at the results. Has all that fear, anger, and grief made you happy, or do you wallow in addiction and misery?

Being willing to clean up the mess you've made of your life will come through the desire for a better way to live, free not only of your addictions, but of all those unexpressed emotions that you mistakenly believed you could blot out, avoid, or escape with addictive behavior. The only way to get forgiveness is by giving it to others.

If you have a problem working up the willing- ness to make amends to those you have harmed, ask the God of your understanding for help. Once you've faced the list, you will have a clear under-standing of your part in things, and who you need to resolve things with. Changing the way we think and behave is the beginning of a clarity which helps us realize the extent of the harm we caused in the past—even as it continues to haunt us in the present.

Once you've said the words out loud to this God of your understanding, ask for the willingness to resolve things with the people you've harmed. This is the start of a process to remove the bur-dens of guilt and shame that may have hardened your heart and kept you from all the wonderful relationships waiting for you in the future.

Recycle

Early on in recovery, you might start to feel as though you are in limbo between the world you knew and a different type of existence. It can be lonely and confusing. If you find yourself wallowing in self-pity, grieving for what was, and fearful of what is to come, it's time to recycle.

Recycling is not merely about old cans, bottles, plastic containers, and newspapers. It's what happens next that's interesting. New things are made from the recycled material—paper, different bottles, shopping bags, even jewelry. Webster's dictionary says to recycle is to "pass through a series of changes or treatment: to alter: to adapt to a new use."

By the time many of us get into recovery, we have pushed away those who care for us because they loved us enough to tell us the truth. Others could no longer participate in our self-destructive lives and pulled away themselves.

Human beings are social animals. We need other people, and when we lose them, even through our own choices, we grieve. Recycling is about altering the way you think and adapting your actions accordingly. If you want a new way of life, a fresh start, it's time to take care of old business. To do that effectively, take out your list of those you have harmed, and go to work.

How do you focus solely on what *you* did, how *you* reacted—and not what the people around you did? Remind yourself that putting things right isn't so much about the other person. It's about clearing away the wreckage of your past so that you might move forward

If you want a new way of life, a fresh start, it's time to take care of old business.

in a happier, healthier way. Whatever the other person's contribution to the situation was, that is between them and their conscience. They get to choose if, or when, they seek recovery.

Beware of temptations. I know some of them well. The first is procrastinating because you assume you know how the other person will react to your apology. You don't know what's in another person's mind and heart. Some of the people I approached who I thought would react badly, didn't; others, who I thought would accept my apology with grace and compassion, didn't. The point is to give them the right to feel, and act, in their truth. They must live with their reaction, not you.

The second temptation is justification—allowing your mind to tell you that the other person did much worse things to you than you did to them, so you don't have owe them an apology. For the recovery process to be successful, you must be able to put aside what others "did" to you. You will continue to carry the burdens of anger and grief—and even though you do not have to face the other person in the mirror each day, you *do* have to face yourself. Justification is usually born of fear, and the only way to overcome fear is to walk through it.

Another temptation, one which I gave into, is the misuse of the process. There was this guy who I had strong feelings for many years before my recovery. I told myself that I wanted to apologize to him, but the truth was that I wanted to hook up with him again, and I'd found the perfect excuse to reconnect. It ended in disaster. When he wasn't buying my crap, I lost my temper and said and did things that actually added to the list of things for which I owed him an apology. Through that experience, I learned to check my motives and make sure I was approaching each person for the right reasons.

The most dangerous temptation is causing more drama or inflicting further harm. This process isn't about martyring ourselves or making ourselves out to be the victim by bringing others into the equation. For instance, it is not acceptable to apologize to someone's wife or husband, telling them you cheated with their spouse. That is for the other person involved to tell them, or not. We can only admit to the things we did to harm another without hurting anyone else or rationalizing it in any way. If it is appropriate, we may need to make restitution. I not only cheated, lied, and manipulated situations, but I had a bad case of sticky fingers. It took me a while, but I attempted to pay back those I could.

There's the rub. Many of the people I'd harmed were dead, some had moved away, others I'd lost touch with, and of course there were those who wanted absolutely nothing more to do with me, and with good reason. My friends in recovery suggested that I take care of the easier ones first. For me, none of them were easy. I decided to take care of the ones that weighed on my mind first. I needed relief if I was going to stay in recovery and release the burden of grief that shackled me to the past.

Letters to the dead were written and burned. I made many visits to cemeteries, apologizing to headstones. I talked to friends and relatives of those who had moved away, and finally attempted to talk to those who had written me off a long time ago. Of course, there were some who I couldn't find or connect with, so I prayed about each situation and told this God of my understanding that I was willing. Over the years, I was amazed to find that many people from my past were put in my path, and I had the opportunity to apologize.

The key here is to go about this process with no expectations. Be honest with yourself about your motives, and take care of *all* the people you have harmed, not just the "easy" ones. Understand that how others react to you is their right. You are doing this to lift the burdens that have been holding you back for years. It may take time, it will take effort, it will be a humbling experience, but at the completion there will be a peace of mind that allows you to lay your head on the pillow at night, close your eyes, and know what it is to sleep like a baby. You have wiped the slate clean. You have recycled yourself into a human being who will not only be of better use to yourself, but to others.

It may take time, it will take effort, it will be a humbling experience, but at the completion there will be a peace of mind that allows you to lay your head on the pillow at night, close your eyes, and know what it is to sleep like a baby.

Balance Sheet

Say you've finished your "G" list. Did you let out a big sigh of relief? Good job! You've faced your demons head on, experienced all those feelings you avoided through your addiction for years, and made things right with others and yourself where and when you could. Now it's time for a better life. But what does that mean?

Years ago I saw a poster that showed a baby chicken just hatched out of an egg. The caption below it said, "What now?"

I have come to understand that feeling. In the first years of my recovery there was a lot of work to be done; every day I woke up with purpose. Although I'd physically buried my children, my mother, and so many others years before, I had to put them to rest, mentally and emotionally. I faced my fears and dealt with the anger and resentments that kept me addicted. Suddenly, it was over. Life was good, and I barely knew how to handle it.

But dear God, I missed the drama that had ruled my very existence for over thirty-five years. It felt as if I'd lost a limb. I'd thrived on extreme highs and lows, even in recovery, for most of my life. The question that kept running through my mind was, "What do calm, peaceful people do with their time, with their thoughts?

Will I be bored to death? Will I be able to cope with all this serenity?" An anti-climatic feeling overwhelmed me.

> What do calm, peaceful people do with their time, with their thoughts?

As time passed, as I became accustomed to a peaceful life, I finally understood that everyday life had enough drama to keep me interested and challenged, and I began to relax. I honestly thought I had it made. But as life has a way of doing, it threw me a curve ball. Suddenly things out of my control were beginning to happen. Someone I cared deeply for was dying; people weren't doing what I thought they should do; a serious illness was plaguing my body. Net result: old fears crept into my mind, followed closely by anger.

My thoughts wandered to the past, back to the ever-present grief I'd used as an excuse for my inappropriate, self-destructive behavior. What in the world was wrong with me? How did things get out of hand so quickly? Was I setting myself up for a relapse? As those questions entered my mind, fear gripped me. I would not go back to the way I'd lived. But how was I to fix it?

Desperate, I sought out a woman who had been a part of my support system before I pulled away from it, telling myself I was clearly too busy with my new life, and that I really didn't need those people (or her) any longer. We met up, and she was full of questions: Had I made my lists, taken care of the people I'd harmed, made a spiritual connection? When I answered yes to those questions, she had one more for me. She said, "What are you doing now?"

Now? Incensed and appalled by the question, I could feel that old familiar rage building inside me. I'd done everything that had been suggested to me by others in recovery. It was hard, but I did it. I had relived excruciating times in my life. I'd cried a river of tears, finally allowing myself to feel what I'd been avoiding for years. I'd even taken responsibility for the hurt I'd caused others, going so far as to apologize to many who had hurt me. What more would I have to do? I snapped at the woman, telling her that I'd already been through quite enough for one lifetime.

She smiled. Smiled! Then, she repeated the question, "What are you doing now?"

Now, today, is the most important time in your life. It is all you really have. Holding on to the past or dreaming of the future only steals away this very moment, this day, and the ability to live life to the fullest. I knew that, had heard it so many times, but I was not practicing it. I wasn't taking care of business on a daily basis. I'd been so busy with my new husband, home, and work, that I forgot what kept me sane and functioning without my addictions. I'd allowed my life to become big, dramatic, and chaotic, and that little grief devil was whispering in my ear again.

Now, today, is the most important time in your life.

What are you doing now? I can tell you what I'm doing. Each day, I do a mental balance sheet that tells me exactly where I am, what I'm doing, and what I need to take care of.

When I go to bed at night and find it difficult to sleep, I reevaluate my day.

Did I pray today?

Was I manipulative?

Did I tell a lie?

Did I offend, cheat, or hurt anyone in any way?

Was I judgmental when I could have been compassionate, hateful in thought or deed when I could have acted in a loving way?

When in the wrong, did I promptly admit it and make things right?

The bottom line is: Am I living the way I say I believe to the best of my ability?

Are you living the way you say you believe? If not, then you might be in conflict between what you say and what you do. This can cause frustration, and put you on that slippery slope back to thinking of your grief and considering reclaiming your addiction. If you are doing that mental balance sheet every day, taking care of things when they happen so that they don't build up, you know what it is to live in the moment, not missing the right now, whatever it brings.

If you are doing that mental balance sheet every day, you know what it is to live in the moment.

You never know how much time you have on this earth, so don't let the moments slip by as you agonize over past experiences or fantasize about tomorrow. This moment and this day are yours, and what you do with them is your choice.

Who Loves Ya, Baby?

I gave up on God, but God never gave up on me. I can't imagine the amount of love and compassion it took for him to believe I had any potential as I floundered, punished myself and others, and continually blamed him—all the while denying his existence. I only acknowledged the possibility of a God when it was convenient for me.

Except for a short period of time when my mother was facing a serious illness, I never had any spiritual beliefs. During my brief encounter with religion, the only thing I took away from the experience was that I would never be able to live up to what the minister said. God would smite me for sure, and when I died, I would live in hell and burn for an eternity. Maybe Grandma Alma was right when she said I was a devil child.

I wanted to be good, but it never seemed to work out that way. No matter what I attempted to do, it was never good enough. Since it didn't seem to matter, after a while I couldn't distinguish the difference between right and wrong. As I aged, my life became about survival, and doing whatever I thought I had to do to that end. I knew that if there were a God out there, he wasn't going to save me from my life and the horrible things that were beginning to happen to me.

From time to time, when my circumstances were dire, I secretly tried praying. I wanted to believe it would work, that my babies and my mother wouldn't die, that my husband at the time would stop hitting me, that I'd find a way to feed myself and my son, that we would have a warm, safe place to sleep at night. But death took those I loved. I had to do some disgusting things to fill our bellies and find a place to sleep. I never felt safe. Finally, I gave up on prayer. I gave up on a God who I thought allowed these things to happen in my life.

While I was active in my addictions, I only acknowledged the possibility of a God when it was convenient for me.

Like a pit bull, I grabbed hold of my grief and refused to turn it loose, using it to excuse my behavior and justify my addictions. When my oldest son was killed at age fifteen, I thought my life was over. There was nothing or nobody left for me. The pain of love and loss turned my heart to stone, my thoughts to rage, and all I had left was my fear, grief, and addictions...or so I thought.

I thought about suicide all the time. But I was afraid that I might screw it up and end up a vegetable. And I doubted that there was another life waiting for me on the other side, if there was indeed another side. All that kept me breathing, but not really alive.

Exhaustion was the catalyst that took me to a recovery program. I was just so tired—tired of being sad and lonely, tired of fighting everything and everyone, and tired of living with my strange thoughts that would surely lead me to insanity. The day my mom shot herself, she said those very words. I asked her what was wrong, and she said, "I'm just tired." I didn't understand her then, but I came to understand what she meant.

Do you know that feeling of being so weary with life that you simply want to step out of it?

Do your days feel like an exercise in frustration and misery?

Do you wake up with a feeling of dread?

Are you using an addiction to escape your feelings?

There is a way of stepping out of an unhappy existence without stepping out of life entirely. Maybe the solution is to step back into life, facing it head on. It's one thing to let go of whatever addiction is affecting you in a negative way, but it's an entirely different prospect to run from those things that caused you to seek out an escape: anger and grief. Facing them will require two things that addicts fear most: trust and love.

The people who were supposed to love and protect me hurt me, left me, and died, and they taught me early in life that to love another person was to set myself up for disappointment and pain. Years ago, there was a detective drama on television. This bald-headed detective named Kojak, who always had a lollipop hanging out of his mouth, would say, "Who loves ya, baby?" Every time I heard him say that I could feel a lump rise in my throat, and I'd have to fight back the tears. I had no idea what it meant to feel loved, or to trust my heart to another human being. I told myself that I had been beaten and bruised too many times—no one would ever get close enough to touch me again.

How's your heart? Has it been abused? Have you built a cage of fear around it? Do you use anger and addiction to keep others at arm's length to protect it? The problem is that although those things might work to keep others out, they also keep you in. As long as your heart is locked in, you will know a loneliness that can never be filled with any addiction.

To be happy, healthy human beings, we need love as much as we need air to breathe, water to quench our thirst, and food to nourish our bodies. Overcoming past painful experiences will mean learning to trust again. I don't know about you, but for me it took divine intervention.

There came a time in my recovery when not indulging in my addictions wasn't enough. Physically I felt better. I had found some mental clarity. But spiritually, I was bankrupt. I was trying to be spiritual, to make that daily connection with a God, but I didn't feel it. I knew I was in danger of a relapse. As soon as I was put in a painful situation, I found myself at a crossroad. It was either go backwards or go forward. I knew what was behind me. To move forward would mean total surrender. I fell to my knees.

I don't know much about the bible, but I remember the story of Moses. On that day I think

I felt what he must have felt when he collapsed in the desert and surrendered. In that instant, I knew what it felt like to be surrounded by real love, to feel safe, to know that I would never have to walk alone again. It wasn't one of those feelings I would only experience once, because I continued the same practice every day. Every day, I got to feel it all over again.

Great events came to pass. I married the love of my life, the man I had been afraid to be with for eighteen years. I had a real home. I started my own costume rental business. I felt like a *real* person for the first time in my life.

I was soon handed a life lesson that I hope I never forget. Although I didn't do it consciously, somewhere in my sick little mind I decided that I'd paid my dues. I didn't need to go to meetings, to get down on my knees every morning and surrender myself. I was fine, fine, fine.

Addicts in recovery know to be extra cautious when something bad happens, but what about when things are going well? During peaceful times, recovery and spirituality often begin to take a back seat to ego. Once we have "arrived," we may think there is no need to continue doing those things that worked to bring us to a better life. Our minds may tell us that we are doing it on our own…that all we needed to do was let go of the addiction. This way of thinking can be a big mistake.

Grief is a funny thing. Even if you've worked through the feelings of loss, the memories remain, and they can be pulled out when, or if, you need the excuse of self-pity to allow you to return to your addiction or pick up a new one. That's what happened to me when I stopped doing those daily things that not only kept me in recovery, but kept me happy and grateful for the life I'd been given. Suddenly I thought I could indulge again, but this time I'd be able to handle it because I had such a good life. Thank goodness I realized where my thoughts had wandered before it was too late.

I'd made countless excuses for not praying and meditating in the mornings. I was busy. I was tired. I slept in. I had to get breakfast on the table. I had to let the dogs out. Pretty soon I didn't even bother with excuses. I simply didn't do it—and I was in trouble. What I discovered was that we make time for what is important. All I had to do was get up an hour earlier in the morning for the prayer and meditation that reminded me each day of who I was and what I was supposed to be doing.

Prayer and meditation is not some automated habit for me. It is serious business, and the quality of my life depends on it. I talk to the God of my understanding as if he were my best friend, because he is. I believe that no matter what happens—and life will keep happening—it is always for my best in the long run. When I listen for direction during meditation, I always find a solution to whatever problem I might be facing. It's not always an easy solution, but it's always the best.

God healed my heart, which allows me to entrust it to others, to open myself to loving and being loved without fear. There is no room left for anger and resentment, and all the grief I've known has been tucked away where it cannot affect my choices today. I am not perfect, but as long as I make that conscious connection to the God of my understanding each day through prayer, I am the best me I can be.

There was the life I thought I'd live out in misery over my grief, isolated from the world around me, filled with fear and anger. Then there is the wonderful life I have been given since that first moment of surrender. Imagine what might be waiting for you when you are willing to open the door, to trust a God of your understanding to show you the way. Like me, I believe you will be amazed. The world is waiting for you when you are ready.

Today, when I think of the television detective saying, "Who loves ya, baby?" I know who loves me.

Good Grief

It hits us like a big wave. We fear that it will swallow us up. We never know when the next wave will come, but sooner or later it will wash over us again. Will this be the one that takes us down, that is so strong that we can't fight it back and survive?

This is grief. It is a surge of emotion so powerful that we don't know what to do with it. I know what it feels like to be swamped by grief, to live in fear of what will trigger the next wave. It could be a word, sound, smell, taste, or even a date on the calendar. At times, for me, it has been a scene on a television program, a story in the newspaper, or even a commercial.

> Grief is a powerful surge of emotion that can be triggered by anything.

For most of my life, normality was one of my greatest triggers. It was as if I was looking at the real world through a window. There were families sitting down to a meal together, celebrating holidays, having picnics, treating each other in a loving way. That wasn't my life, so I always felt like I was on the outside looking in.

Once I was in recovery from my addictions, I wanted so badly to be a better person. I tried to live with joy in my heart, gratitude for each new day. I sought to live within the bounds of humanity; I tried to be perfect. When I allowed other feelings to intrude, I felt like I wasn't doing it right, that I shouldn't feel whatever I was feeling. That brought on guilt and shame, even anger at myself for failing yet again.

I believed that I had to love everyone. The truth was that I didn't even come close to loving everyone. In fact, there were many people who I didn't even like. When things didn't go my way, I felt anger creep in. Some days I focused on the future, fearful of what was to come. Waves of sadness over past losses gripped my heart. I became consumed by the question, "What is wrong with me?"

My life became a paradox. I was addiction-free and had found faith in a God of my understanding, so why was I still having these feelings? Finally, I opened that particular can of worms to a trusted friend. She said, "I wondered when you were going to give yourself permission to be a normal human being."

Acceptance is agreeing with what already is. I'd closed myself off from the world using anger and addiction as my shield. Those were the facts. Fearful of being devoured by grief, I put on a tough, stoic mask for the world to see. But all my unexpressed emotions were nearly devouring me with grief from the inside out. It was one thing to accept the truth of what actually happened to me, and an entirely different thing to accept my feelings about what happened.

> Acceptance is agreeing with what already is.

I don't know when it became the norm for humans to be stoic when grieving, but I know in my case that it didn't work well. Many of us, including myself, put on a brave face, get through the initial shock, and then spend years attempting to drown, numb, or distract our real feelings. Can you imagine what a profound relief it would be to have a screaming fit, letting the huge explosion of emotion out?

A dear friend of mine, who happened to be a psychologist, gave me a way to do exactly that. He suggested that when I felt a wave of grief wash over me, I go to my bedroom, set my alarm clock for half an hour, and let it all out. So I did what he told me. I wept. I punched pillows. I screamed out every thought and question in my mind. I cursed. I stomped. I yelled at God, crying out,

"Why…why…why?" When my alarm buzzed, I stopped. If you had seen me, you would have thought I'd lost my mind, but it worked—and it still works.

I had mistakenly believed that, in my recovery, I should no longer feel grief or know anger and fear. I wondered how I could claim to have faith, know joy, be spiritual, and still feel those things. It was like I was setting myself above my humanity. I am a human being, and throughout my life I will experience every human emotion.

To deal with grief in a healthy way is to participate in the expression of your true feelings.

The key word here is "experience." Experience denotes participation. To deal with grief in a healthy way is to participate in the expression of your true feelings.

Do you do that to yourself—say to yourself that you should be better than you are, put unrealistic expectations on yourself and feel badly when you don't live up to them?

Do you fight your true feelings about your losses?

Wouldn't you like to let loose, say what's really on your mind, what lives in your heart?

Are you afraid your God won't like you any-more if you say it out loud?

Here's a newsflash…you are not perfect either. The good news is that you don't have to be.

A wise man once told me not to confuse the God of my understanding with human beings. He said, "God doesn't expect any more of you than you are willing to give." He assured me that I could love the human race as a whole, but I didn't have to like every individual. Another friend told me that it is easy to love the lovable, and it's the same with faith. It's easy to have faith when things go the way I think they should. The true test of faith is when we are challenged through loss and continue to hold on to our belief that whatever we are going through is a part of our path.

Grief is a part of the human experience. It serves a purpose in our lives. For many, it stops us in our tracks, causing us to re-evaluate our priorities. For some, it brings us to a crossroad where we are forced to make a choice about which direction to take. Some of us, like me, choose the path of denial, live in fear, and express ourselves through anger and addiction. But the grief that changed our path waits patiently for us to face it and work our way back, for us to realize that we have learned a great life lesson. So, I say, "Good grief."

You might be thinking, wasn't it the pain of grief that drove me to become an addict? It was the choice I made not to participate honestly in my feelings about what happened to me that drove me to addictions. But it was the same pain that brought me to my knees the day I surrendered to a God of my understanding. It was the same pain that brought me to recovery. A woman once said to me, "If one thing had happened differently in your life, you wouldn't be here today, the person you are, doing what you're doing." The addiction is a response to pain—a response to try to deny my feelings, and the pain of the addiction, led to my choice to deal with the grief and my choice for recovery.

As I continue down my path, I will know grief again. The difference is that today I recognize it for what it is: a moment of choice that can alter my life.

The great life lesson that I took from overcoming grief is that there is a reason for everything under the sun, and that through my faith in believing in something of which I have no understanding, there is a purpose for me.

I am no longer a wandering addict, but a person I never thought I could be, doing things that I was completely incapable of doing on my own. As I continue down my path, I will know grief again. The difference is that today I recognize it for what it is: a moment of choice that can alter my life. When that choice comes, you can find me in my bedroom, alarm clock set, having a cathartic fit until I get it all out. I am. I feel. I heal.

All or Nothing

Return to your addiction, or pick up a new addiction, and those old familiar feelings of fear, anger, and grief that you used to justify your actions will jump on the bandwagon shortly after. The past is not gone—you have not altered what happened before—all you have done is change your perspective. If you allow new fears, anger, and grief to enter your life in recovery, addiction is right around the corner.

Just as you exercise your body to achieve physical fitness, your spiritual fitness is contingent on daily prayer and meditation.

Beware of arrogance and apathy. Those who become arrogant convince themselves that they have somehow accomplished recovery on their own, when the truth is that they are the ones who got themselves in the mess in the first place. One of the definitions in Webster's Dictionary for apathy is "spiritless." Just as you exercise your body to achieve physical fitness, your spiritual fitness is contingent on daily prayer and meditation. Spiritual apathy will leave you sluggish and dispirited.

If you are honestly spiritual, how can you know your God's will for you unless you ask through prayer and listen through meditation? This spiritual thing isn't something you do once. You must return to it once a day, because each day is as important as any other. You never know what the new day will bring. Life can change in an instant and if you are not spiritually sound, everything you've worked so diligently towards can go out the window.

Most of us will face a crisis of faith at some point in our recovery. We might question what's happening in our lives, and it's asking a lot of a human being to believe that everything is for the best when it seems so wrong. However, if you are on path, that's what will be required of you if you are to continue the journey. I certainly experienced challenges and questioning during my recovery, and I worked with many others in similar situations.

Among the most difficult things we face in recovery are those pesky emotions that continue to crop up. We no longer have a buffer of addiction to avoid the feelings—no way to run, no distractions. It can make us feel naked, vulnerable, and tempted to step backwards to those old behaviors.

I know that's how I felt—my life was finally going well, and then the rug was jerked out under me.

I was flying high. Life was better than I could have dreamed. I'd married the love of my life, finally had a real home and a car that ran every day. I didn't have to worry about having enough to eat or that anyone would hit me. But most importantly, I *liked* the person I'd become. I'd realized a dream of starting my own business, and it was thriving. I assumed that I'd be doing that kind of work for the rest of my life. Not!

I became physically ill. For months the illness progressed with no diagnosis until I believed it would lead to my death. Fear set in, followed quickly by anger, then grief. I grieved for the limitations that were taking away everything I'd worked so hard to build and achieve. I realized I was at a crossroad—that the decision I made at that time would affect the rest of the time I had left. I can't say that I didn't want immediate relief, that I didn't struggle with the decision. But ultimately I chose to believe. Once I made the choice, even though I was still very sick, things began to change. I started to focus on what I *could* do instead of what I couldn't do. I stopped fearing what might lie ahead, living in the moments of my life. As I let go of the grief over my limitations, I had no reason to feel anger.

The specific disease doesn't really matter. Many people will have various diseases, get injured in accidents, become victims of crimes, or have to watch as someone they love experiences the same things, or dies. What is important is how we deal with those situations. I was fortunate that my disease was diagnosed, that doctors treated me, and that I survived—but I'd already made my peace with the disease. Through prayer and meditation I came to understand that whatever happened would be okay. I'd done my part, the doctors had done theirs, and the rest was up to the God of my understanding.

As I walk through my life today, I am never alone. My God walks with me through every challenge, great and small, as long as I make the effort to stay connected through prayer and meditation. I spent a lot of years crippled and angry by the past, fearful of the future and afraid to let go of my grief and the self-destructive addictions that were ruining my life. Now, I treasure the day, knowing each moment can bring wonder and joy. No matter

> As I walk through life today, I am never alone.

what is going on outside of me, it's okay for me to hold on to that joy.

Many years ago in my early recovery, a man told me that the day would come when I would be able to be the voice of joy. I couldn't believe that would ever happen, but here I am. I always wondered what purpose I served in this world. Now I know. I get to be the voice of joy, of hope, not only for those new to recovery, but for everyone who crosses my path. I can share a smile, lend a helping hand, or share my experience, strength, and hope with others. It brings me a joy I never knew existed.

If you truly want to know your purpose, all you need to do is ask the God of your understanding, listen with your heart instead of your ears, and believe not what your brain tells you, but what your soul knows.

Do you do that—wonder why you're here, what the point is? I believe that every person is here for a reason. Otherwise they wouldn't be here. If you truly want to know the reason, your purpose, all you need to do is ask the God of your understanding, listen with your heart instead of your ears, and believe not what your brain tells you, but what your soul knows.

Letting Go

"Just let it go!" I recently heard a therapist on a television show nearly shout that out to a lady. I've heard the same phrase used in treatment centers, from some in 12-step meetings, and have been told by people who work with others that it's what they say in response to a person who continually dwells on a particular event in his or her life. Do they honestly believe that if people who have lived through crisis, trauma, tragedy, and loss could "just let it go"—if it were that simple—they would be exposing their problem on national television, spending tens of thousands of dollars in treatment, or going to meeting after meeting, asking for help?

Letting go is a process, and the time and effort required is as individual as each person. For many years I wrapped myself in an invisible security blanket woven by grief and fear so that others wouldn't know me or see the pain that lived inside, day in and day out. I attempted to numb and distract the pain with addictions, and used anger to keep others from getting too close. I was like a small child holding on to her blanket for dear life. It may have been old, ragged, and dirty, but somehow it made me feel secure in a frightening world. You don't just rip that blanket out of a child's hands—or an addict's hands. It can be devastating. And we don't just let it go.

When using that phrase with another person, you might as well say to them, "You are defective. There is something wrong with you if you can't just let it go. Other people get through it. It's time." How can anyone else know what you're going through, when the right time is, when you've been cloaked in your invisible blanket for so long? The blanket has four corners, representing fear, anger, grief, and addiction. When you become ready to begin the process of letting go, which corner do you let go of first?

(Hint: It doesn't really matter because it is a process.)

Fear, Anger, Grief, Addiction

Fear

The great boogeyman, fear of the unknown, is what keeps us trapped in lives of misery. Like children, we find a familiar place we believe to be safe and predictable, pull the covers over our heads, and think life can't get us. The truth is that life doesn't have to get us, because we are doing such a good job of it ourselves.

You've seen it, perhaps experienced it. There are those who stay in abusive relationships or dead-end jobs that they hate; others who continue to return to destructive behavior and addictions; and runners, who flit here and there, doing this and that, in the vain belief that they can outrun the reality that is their life. These people cling to the familiar, even though it's an unhappy existence, because they fear what "might" be out there in the great unknown.

Often it isn't until our misery becomes greater than our fear that we make the decision to come out of hiding and face the boogeyman head on. When we decide that what might be out there can't be any worse than the here and now, we make the leap, only to end up repeating a similar scenario. That means we haven't dealt with the issue—we've simply dragged it along with us.

Changing your perception of time is the answer to the challenge of fear. It may sound trite to tell you to live in each moment as if it is your last, but the truth is that it is possible. I recall the first time I actually gave that idea some thought. I wondered, "How does one do that? I don't mean think about it, but put it into practice. How can that work? Am I not doing my job as a responsible person if I'm not worrying about things?"

If you wonder how well you are living in the moments of your life, make a list of all the unchangeable things you worried about today. Did those worrying moments keep you from enjoying your family and friends, take anything away from your peace of mind, or give you a restless night? Did your worrying change one thing? Yes, it robbed you of being present in a moment you will never be able to recapture.

What is our goal, after all, but to be happy? You noticed I didn't say the pursuit of happiness. To pursue means to chase, to follow, to go after something. As long as you pursue it, it will evade you. It may be right in front of your nose, but as long as you are looking down the road, trying to attain happiness, you won't recognize it.

Even though we may fear the unknown, we often believe that there is time to take care of things, to make the changes that will bring us happiness. The time is now, my friend. It's all you really have. You have a choice to be present in each moment or to toss them away in the vain hope that there will be time later. What if later never comes? I heard that. You thought, "Then I won't have to worry about things anymore." What if that isn't true? What if there's another existence after this one, and you must continue facing the life lessons you didn't learn this time around?

As long as you live in the now, what is there to fear? You have been given this very moment to do whatever you choose. There is joy to be found in the smallest things. There is always something for which to be grateful. I believe that something good can come out of even the most tragic events.

There is joy to be found in the smallest things. There is always something for which to be grateful. I believe that something good can come out of even the most tragic events. Courage isn't about being fearless, but about walking through the fear at the moment it occurs. Fear is optional. Happiness is a choice we make each day. The only way to vanquish the boogeyman is to not believe it exists. As long as there is no tomorrow, all we have is today...this moment...now.

You can embrace each dawning of the sun with anticipation of new people, experiences, and feelings; hold joy in your heart no matter what happens; or pull the covers over your head, tremble in fear, and miss out on all that this life has to offer. It's your choice.

Anger

Anger serves several purposes. You've probably heard someone say, "He's out of control," when speaking of an angry person. In actuality, that person may be using anger in an attempt to control others or a situation. I grew up with an angry, controlling stepfather. It was like living in a minefield, always having to watch my step to avoid the next explosion. Each time an explosion happened it blew off a piece of me. I learned to hate; to live in my own anger.

As intimidated as I was by my stepfather in my childhood, as I look back today, I no longer hate him. I feel sad for him. I don't know what happened to him that made him feel as if he had no control over his life, that made it so important to control everything and everyone around him, but whatever it was left a huge open sore in him that never healed. Regardless, I carried my anger toward him into my adult years. It became the catalyst for rebellion against authority and justification for self-pity that showed itself in anger and addictions.

"The squeaky wheel gets oiled" is an old adage. It means that he who yells the loudest gets attention. It didn't take me long to figure out that if I wanted attention, all I had to do was go into a rage. People notice that. They become interested, wanting to know what's wrong or if they can do something to help. It's not that much different than a screaming baby who is trying to get her needs met. When it worked, raging gave me a feeling of power.

When we feel invisible, unimportant, or powerless, anger becomes a manipulation tool that we use to assuage those feelings. It's like crying out, "Somebody see me, hear me, know that what I'm saying without words is important. Does anyone care? I'm important too! Help me!" It's a catch-22; anger keeps us from using the real words we need to use to get our needs met, which leads to even more anger.

For addicts, anger is the best hiding place for those feelings that make them vulnerable and uncomfortable. If they could deal with reality and the expression of their true feelings, they wouldn't need to escape through addictions. I understand this scenario so well. While living as an addict, no matter what happened, I went directly to anger and responded accordingly. Believe me when I tell you that if your comfort zone is anger, you can always find something to be pissed about, and someone else to blame.

As long as addicts can blame others and keep the focus off of themselves, they don't have to take responsibility for anything. When raging, two of their favorite words to use are "if" and "but." I've used those words a lot myself, and when working with other addicts, I listen for them. They tell me that those people are still filled with anger—they are blaming anything or anyone outside themselves. As soon as I hear, "If she hadn't done that, I wouldn't have gone out to drink, drug, gamble, or whatever," or "Yes, but he or she did this or that," or "Yes, but you don't know what happened to me," red flags immediately go up.

Letting go of anger will require self-focus and taking responsibility for your actions, no matter what is going on around you. It's not as if you won't get angry in recovery. But it's how you process it and act on it that is important. There may be times when you can't help how you feel, but you always have a choice of what you do.

Two people are required for an argument. What if one person walks away, refusing to participate? It's more important to be happy than it is to be right. People believe what they choose to believe, and nothing you can say or do will change that. If you expect others to respect your beliefs, you must allow them the same respect. When you can do that, it eliminates the power struggle that we see so often in love, friend, and work relationships. If you get off on the feeling of having power over others, you need to take a look at what is going on with you. Why do you need to do that to feel good about yourself?

We have a part in every personal encounter or situation. It's important to scrutinize what we contributed to each encounter or situation, positive or negative. It's too easy to place the blame elsewhere, and to hide our true feelings behind anger.

One day a girlfriend of mine said something that hurt my feelings. Instead of telling her that, I got mad. From that moment on, until I confronted the situation and expressed how I felt, the anger lived and grew inside me. When I saw her, it was always in the back of my mind. I found myself picking at her in the ridiculous belief that if I could hurt her back, we'd be even. When I realized what I was doing, I came to the understanding that to let it go on would simply escalate the situation, which could eventually destroy the friendship. To my amazement, she was appalled at herself for having said what she did, and she apologized to me immediately. I kicked myself for the time wasted and the bad feelings I'd put myself through for so long.

> When you are angry with another person, they own you. They are in control of your time, feelings, and actions.

When I finally let go of my anger, I remembered some things that others in recovery told me. One is that when you are angry with another person, they own you. They are in control of your time, feelings, and actions. Why would I let anyone live rent-free in my head? They take up space in my mind that could be used for more positive, productive thoughts.

Using anger as a manipulation tool for gaining attention is about keeping the drama alive in your life, which brings us to the topic of grief.

Grief

Grieving over loss is normal. Holding on to that grief for years, as I did, and using it for attention, to manipulate others, and as the ultimate excuse for bizarre behavior, is not. In the past there were rules for grieving the loss of a loved one. People cloaked themselves in black and did not attend social functions for the first year. That was probably a good idea, but what did they do with sorrow over other losses? I imagine we aren't all that different than we are today.

Grief is the last stronghold of addicts. Letting go of grief is giving up justification for self-involvement and self-pity—the perfect excuse to step backwards into addiction when the road to recovery gets bumpy. And, it's legitimate. Pain over loss is real, it hurts, many times crushing the dreams and expectations of the future. Even after the initial anger over a loss passes, a simmering resentment can settle in.

> Grief is the last stronghold of addicts.

It's not easy to overcome grief in recovery, not having an addiction as a buffer. When I was grieving, I wished I could simply go through withdrawal like I did from booze and drugs, and get on with my recovery one day at a time.

However, I'd only been a full-blown addict for eighteen years, and I'd been grieving my entire life. It was almost as if I'd grown an extra limb, had gotten used to using it, and couldn't imagine life without it.

I'd lost a lot of people to death in my life, but believe me when I tell you I'd been wallowing in self-pity from grief for years before anyone died, or before I picked up the first pill and drink. I compared my life to others'—and it never measured up. My life was not what I expected, what I thought I deserved. I was not who I wanted to be. And in my grief I blamed everyone and everything for my plight. I told myself it couldn't be my fault. Perhaps I was right. Many of the things that happened to me in childhood were not my fault, but the choices I made later were.

Two things that helped me let go of my grief: compassionate forgiveness and taking responsibility. To achieve true forgiveness means to completely let go of whatever happened—it doesn't mean that you store the old situation and feelings up for later use in case you need them. To do that will require compassion for those from your past.

I found it interesting that after getting into recovery and working with new people—listening to their stories, many of which involved how they hurt others in ways similar to how I was hurt—I felt compassion for them. As I listened to their stories unfold, I got a clearer understanding of what happened to them to bring on the addiction and behavior. I learned to empathize. I recognized that I had no idea what happened to those people who hurt me. I knew nothing about them, judging them without all the information I needed to see them clearly.

What if, like me, grief had a hold on them, and they reacted to life and people accordingly? What if their actions had nothing to do with me? Did that mean I wasn't stupid, ugly, and unlovable? When I realized this, I don't know if I was stunned or relieved. I'd wasted a lot time and energy blaming them, hating myself, chasing one after another, and never finding any lasting relief. With that realization, I began to understand what it meant to take responsibility for my own choices and actions.

Imagine two people from nearly parallel tragic backgrounds. One rises above his past and attributes his success in life to having lived through the tragedies that made him stronger. The other sinks to the bottom of the barrel and blames his lack of success on the past. What is it that makes them different? It's that when they become old enough to make their own choices, they choose different paths. Forgiving others and letting go of grief are conscious choices.

It sounds easy enough, but for those of us who have made the choice to hang on to our grief, it will take some work to stop it. How do you do that? I acted as an investigator, asking questions of those in my life in order to have a better understanding of where they came from. I was absolutely amazed at my discoveries. Through my investigation, I opened myself up to the truth, and it became clear to me that the people who wronged me in life were not bad people, but sad people who made poor choices. Those choices involved using their grief as an excuse to live in fear, anger, and addictions, lashing out at the world and its inhabitants. I just happened to be close by. And I followed in their footsteps.

It's much easier to hold a grudge against a bad person than it is to hate a sad person. That's when the ability to empathize comes into play. Empathy involves vicariously putting yourself in another person's shoes, imagining what he or she might have been feeling, and how those feelings might have affected his or her choices. It doesn't mean we have to get re-involved in the lives of those who hurt us, but it gives us a way to release our grief and forgive them.

As you learn to feel empathy, compassion, and forgiveness for others, you will find those things for yourself. You will let go of grief over the poor choices you've made in the past and know that each day is an opportunity for better choices. Even when things happen that are out of your control, you have a choice of how to act, and are responsible for the results of that choice. Choose wisely, because the life it will affect will be your own.

Addiction

Anyone can stop an addiction. The trick is to *stay* stopped. To do that it will be necessary to change not only your behavior, but your way of thinking. It's been said around recovery programs that if you sit in a barbershop long enough, you'll get a haircut. You might think that means that drunks should stay out of bars, gamblers out of casinos, overeaters out of bakeries, and so on. Avoiding past triggers makes sense, but staying in recovery also means finding a way to stay out of your old way of thinking. The longer you hold on to that old mindset, the closer you come to getting a mental haircut.

Which comes first—letting go of the addiction, or the insane thinking that goes along with addictive behavior? It will be essential to remove the addiction first. It's pretty much impossible to think clearly when your mind is sidetracked with an obsession, busy finding excuses, justifications, and rationalizations. To maintain an addiction is work, and it will be work to let go of it.

Some people believe it doesn't matter where your addiction came from, and that delving into the past will only bring you sorrow. There's no doubt that it will—as long as you attempt to ignore the reasons, your mind will surely cause you to return to the addiction or pick up a new one. For real addicts, as long as the reasons for their addiction remain, so does the need to escape.

You may believe you can escape your true feelings about your past—what was done to you, your choices and actions, and the effect they've had on you and those close to you. But if what you desire is lasting recovery, there is no escape. Recovery is not a walk in the park. It's a triathlon, and to make it to the end, you'll have to push through the pain. As any athlete will tell you, you must prepare yourself for endurance. Stopping your addictive behavior will prepare you for what is to come. Then, you will face the "Big 3": fear, anger, and grief.

Recovery is not a walk in the park. It's a triathlon, and to make it to the end, you'll have to push through the pain.

There is a difference between letting go of an addiction and living in recovery. Letting go of an addiction is a day-to-day thing, whereas living in recovery from addiction is a commitment to a lifetime proposition. Addictions are like old lovers waiting for your return. The temptation is great, which accounts for so many relapses. Yes, relapse is a choice. It's been called a "slip," but all "slip" means is that sobriety lost its priority.

Life, with all its ups and downs, will keep happening whether you are in recovery or not. How willing you are to deal with the old baggage you brought with you into recovery, remaining aware of the reality of what you're thinking and feeling, will be essential for a lasting recovery. Recovery doesn't promise you that you won't feel sorrow when there is tragedy and loss, but if you don't own your feelings of grief, grief will own you. This doesn't mean that you will never get angry at an injustice, but there are constructive ways to express that anger. Internalized, anger will build into a great drama and show itself in unhealthy ways. Recovery can be fraught with new fears of facing life addiction-free. There is no way around fear except straight through it, and each time you stare it down, you will be stronger for the next time.

Letting go of the addictive behavior is the tip of the iceberg. Learning to think, feel, and live in recovery after the freedom from addiction will ask so much more from you. Opening your mind to new concepts, being willing to be brutally honest with yourself and others, and making the efforts it will take to change may not be easy. But if what you are seeking is lasting peace and happiness, what you put into it is what you'll get out of it.

Celebrate

How do you feel when you encounter cheerful, happy people who laugh a lot and seem to find some good even in the worst of circumstances? I can recall what my reaction to these people was in the past. I would stick my finger in my mouth and act as if I was gagging. I know now that that's how I demeaned anything I didn't understand and believed I couldn't attain. I envied them, though I would never admit it. Lost in a sea of grief and misery, I considered them a constant reminder of everything I would never be.

Although the particulars may be different, we all go through loss, and have to deal with fear, anger, and grief in our lifetime. Why is it that some people trudge through life dragging their feet in the sand, exhausted and unhappy, and others seem to skip through their lives with a smile? I've come to believe it is a matter of perspective. You may not be able to change your circumstances, but you can learn to see things in a healthier way.

When I lost my infant babies, buried my mother who'd taken her own life, went through one bad relationship after another, and indulged in addictions, there was one thing that kept me going. It was my oldest son, Jon. He was beautiful, healthy, smart, and funny, and he loved me beyond reason. Everyone else had pretty much written me off as a lost cause, but he loved me unconditionally. Then, at age fifteen, he was killed.

His death was the catalyst that after a few years brought me to a hard bottom with my addictions. My options at that point were to kill myself, be put away in an institution, or find a recovery program. Since I had a great fear of ever being locked up again, and apparently wasn't ready to give up my life entirely, I figured the recovery thing was worth a try. I ended up in a 12-step program.

Around the meetings, I heard that we addicts weren't bad people trying to be good, but sick people trying to get well.

As I struggled through the steps, I listened to others who'd been down the path that loomed ahead of me. I finally found a God of my understanding in my life. My perception of the life I'd lived, and the choices in front of me, changed. Around the meetings, I heard that we addicts weren't bad people trying to be good, but sick people trying to get well. You can't imagine what relief that gave me. All my life I thought I was a bad seed and there was no hope for me. Suddenly, there was a glimmer of hope; a small flame ignited in me that maybe I could honestly change.

As time passed and I stayed clean and sober, the fog began to lift in my mind. There were actual moments of clarity. In those moments, the realization of the work ahead, of what it would mean to face my fear, deal with my anger, and resolve the grief that had embedded itself so deeply in me, became almost overwhelming. But I was told I only had to do it one day at a time, that I had the rest of my life to work on it, and that all I had to do was the best I could each day, not comparing my best to anyone else's best. One person said, "This is not a competition, there are no medals, but if you do this thing, amazing events will take place in your life."

I stuck it out. I did the work. Amazing events have taken place in my life. One of those amazing things is that I learned to *celebrate* life on a daily basis. In the past, when those traumatic dates rolled around, and I had a lot of them, I would get depressed, filled with self-pity and anger, and indulge in one addiction after another. I wouldn't wait for the actual date to get there, but began my grieving a month or two ahead, which took me through the entire year. Then I'd start over again. In recovery I celebrate the moments of my life...all of them, because I know that it took every experience to bring me to the person I am today, to the life I live.

Which brings us back to seeing things differently. I recall dwelling on all the things I would miss in my children's lives because they died, and how it made me feel. In recovery, with the help of sage advice and a spiritual connection, I could clearly see that I'd been blessed. For fifteen years I got to be a mother, to share my life with an extraordinary human being, and if I'd known ahead of time all the pain I would endure when I lost him, I wouldn't have given up one moment of time with him.

For the first half of my life, I had nothing to give anyone. I took everything I could from anyone handy, but it was never enough. My experience, strength, and hope is what I have to give today as I work with those in crisis. I get to counsel those who are grieving, angry, fearful, and addicted by sharing my story, and perhaps giving them that one glimmer of hope that was given to me. This has been one of my greatest gifts. I've come to believe that the God of my understanding

Addiction & Grief

saw something in me that no one else could see, and he had a plan for me.

According to Webster's dictionary, one of the definitions of celebrate is "to honor an occasion." Every day I'm granted through grace is an occasion, and I try to honor it the best that I can. I honor those I've lost by loving fully and completely, with no fear. I honor my past by using it to help others. I honor myself by allowing myself to have the life that the God of my understanding chose for me. I honor you by understanding that just as I have a right to my choices, so do you, and it is not for me to judge.

I often sign my books with phrases like Every Moment Counts, Happiness is a Choice, Live Boldly and Unafraid, or The World Is Waiting for You. I'm sure there are those who think they are phrases authors use to have something to say, but when I write those words, I mean them from the deepest part of my soul. I know for a fact that through feeling what you are feeling when you are feeling it, and then fearlessly letting it go when it becomes a problem, you will discover a life worth celebrating on a daily basis. That is the life I celebrate today, and it's the life I hope for you, too.

Dance on Life

Imagine a huge block party. As you approach, wonderful aromas of cooking food fill your nose and make your mouth water in anticipation. Sounds of vibrant music and laughter waft across the air, enticing you to join in. Closer now, your eyes see people of all sizes and colors moving to the rhythm of the music. Because there is such diversity in the crowd, food, and music, you know it's not about age or race. What do you do? How do you feel? If you are honest, it will tell you where you are in life.

Would you feel compelled to join in, filling your senses with all that is offered, letting your body move uninhibited in sync with the beat as the music flowed around you? Would you stand at the edge of the party to watch others as they indulged in the gaiety? Perhaps you think if you had a few drinks, popped some pills, or smoked a joint you could be the life of the party. Or would you simply stand there, held fast by fear that you didn't belong, but envying those who you believe did? Does that fill you with anger? Who do you blame?

If fear holds you back, it is a symptom of not feeling good enough. If anger builds, it is a substitute feeling that you use to mask your true feelings of sorrow over feeling separate from those around you. If you can only participate under the influence of drugs or alcohol, you are pretending to belong. If you blame others, you are grieving for the person you could have been if not for the failings of those in your life. However, if you jump in, explore new tastes, feel the laughter build and explode from your body, and allow yourself to move with the rhythm of the music, you know what it means to dance on life.

To dance on life is about waking up each day filled with anticipation for what a new day holds.

To dance on life is not only about parties, but about waking up each day filled with anticipation for what a new day holds. It is about being grateful for whatever you have to give back to life, a willingness to experience all things that are presented to you. It is a clear understanding that you will not know great joy unless you have experienced great sorrow, that if you refuse to feel the one you will never know the other.

How do you get that feeling of being a part of it all? Here's something somebody suggested to me: Find a quiet, beautiful place where you feel comfortable. If you are able, throw your head back, raise your arms to the sky, and close your eyes. If you are not physically able, picture this exercise in your mind's eye. Listen to the breath coming in through your nose and leaving through your mouth. Hear the beat of your heart as it pulses through your body, pumping life and giving blood. Now, imagine your heart beating in sync with every other heart in the world.

When you truly achieve this feeling, you will know that for every heartbeat, there is a reason and a season. Fear will be replaced by faith, anger by honesty, grief by joy, and addiction by choice. You will be in possession of the great secret of life, which is that you belong with all of humanity, and we all have something to give when we become willing to jump in, to dance on life instead of waiting on the sidelines until it's all over.

About the Author

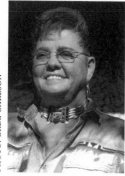

Barb Rogers learned most of her life lessons through great pain and tragedy. After surviving abuse, the death of her children, addiction, and life-threatening illness, she succeeded in finding a new way of life. She became a professional costume designer and founded Broadway Bazaar Costumes. When an illness forced her to give up costume designing, Barb turned to writing. She is the author of three costuming books and several titles on recovery, alcoholism and addiction, and well-being, including *Twenty-Five Words and Keep It Simple and Sane*. Barb Rogers died early in 2011 after a brief final illness.

To Our Readers

Conari Press, an imprint of Red Wheel/Weiser, publishes books on topics ranging from spirituality, personal growth, and relationships to women's issues, parenting, and social issues. Our mission is to publish quality books that will make a difference in people's lives—how we feel about ourselves and how we relate to one another. We value integrity, compassion, and receptivity, both in the books we publish and in the way we do business.

Our readers are our most important resource, and we appreciate your input, suggestions, and ideas about what you would like to see published.

Visit our website at *www.redwheelweiser.com*, where you can subscribe to our newsletters and learn about our upcoming books, exclusive offers, and free downloads.

You can also contact us at *info@redwheel weiser.com*

Conari Press
an imprint of Red Wheel/Weiser, LLC
665 Third Street, Suite 400
San Francisco, CA 94107